In the Meantime

A 28-Day Devotional for Conception Encouragement

KELLI FERGUSON

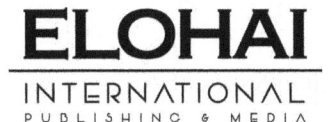

Copyright © 2020
by Kelli Ferguson

All rights reserved. This book or any portion thereof may not be reproduced or used in any manner whatsoever without the express written permission of the publisher except for the use of brief quotations in a book review.

Published by ELOHAI International Publishing & Media
P.O. Box 64402
Virginia Beach, VA 23467
ElohaiPublishing.com

Library of Congress Control Number: 2020915966

ISBN: 978-1-953535-01-6

Printed in the United States of America

To all the women who are paused in their meantime and anticipating a miracle.

Contents

9 Acknowledgments
11 Preface
15 Introduction

WEEK 1

17 Menstrual Phase: And Another One

DAY 1
26 You Better Hustle

DAY 2
29 God's Creative Power: No Assistance Required

DAY 3
32 Check the Receipts!

DAY 4
39 A Dormant Branch

DAY 5
42 Seeds and Sand

DAY 6
45 An Appointed Time

DAY 7
48 Forgiveness = Healing

WEEK 2

53   Follicular Phase: Building Hope

DAY 8
58   God's Authoritative Power: Open and Close

DAY 9
62   Wait Patiently

DAY 10
66   Hearing Aids and Contacts Not Required

DAY 11
70   Having God's Ear

DAY 12
74   Drought Resistant

DAY 13
77   God's Strategic Power: Cracking Open the Jar

DAY 14
81   What's Your Why?

WEEK 3

85   Ovulation Phase: Execution Time!

DAY 15
89   Joined Together

DAY 16
92   The Power of a Praying Mother

DAY 17
96   Hidden Idols

DAY 18
100   Building Muscles

DAY 19
105   Communication Is Key

DAY 20
109   By and By

DAY 21
113   Jailbreak

WEEK 4
117 Luteal Phase: Who's Your Bible Mentor?
DAY 22
125 The Importance of Warming Up
DAY 23
129 Fruitful in the Land of Affliction
DAY 24
133 Healing Tears
DAY 25
137 Feasting in the Famine
DAY 26
140 Restoration of What Was Lost
DAY 27
144 Unexpected Blessings
DAY 28
147 Temporary Space
151 Afterword
153 Reference List
159 About the Author
161 Connect and Share

Acknowledgments

I would like to thank all those who continue to support me through my own meantime, especially Barbara Smith, Georgina Tait, Margie Willis Bond, Sheree Willis Johnson, Valon Thornton, Kimberly Johnson, Chavonne Thompson, Kristina Treadwell, Johnique Billups, and Quiana Broden.

Thanks belong to my crew, Jessica Thornton and Krislynn Thompson, who gave amazing encouragement and feedback throughout the writing process.

Thank you to Tiphani Montgomery whose writing workshop and mentorship has helped to take this devotional from an idea to a reality.

Special thank you to my husband Hugh who encouraged me with back rubs, held me through my tears, and makes the best sounding board anyone could ask for.

Most importantly, thank you to Jesus Christ who is the ultimate Creator and Source of divine inspiration. All glory and honor belong to Him.

Preface

When I was about ten years old, I remember eagerly anticipating the arrival of the new JC Penney catalog. The thick, glossy catalog was filled with hundreds of pages of images that provoked an individual to want, desire, and dream. For me, the inside of the catalog would propel me to a world where fantasies were realized. Once the catalog was in my hands, I would sift through its pages with careful thoughtfulness, looking for exactly the right picture to create my fantasy world. I would take my scissors and spend hours cautiously cutting out each picture that reflected the images of where I wanted life to take me.

    I recall searching through the catalog to find the one black adult female model usually included and imagining her to be me in twenty years. The catalog typically included one or two photos of an entire family unit together—a mom, a dad, a brother, and a sister—that I would use to feed my desire of wanting to have a family of my own someday. Just to clarify, I was blessed beyond measure with the family into which I was born; it's just that the images in the catalog always showed that the beautiful woman was happiest when she was surrounded by her own nuclear family. Even at the age of ten, I knew that my goal in life was to be like the woman in the pictures—well dressed, pressed hair, a handsome husband who was taller than me and wore a high top fade, and a little boy and girl who were always color-coordinated.

A few years later when I was in the eighth grade, I found myself talking out my personal life plan with a friend. We were both supposed to marry our current boyfriends at the age of twenty-three and have our children by the time we were twenty-eight. Ours seemed like a solid plan. We were best friends; the guys were best friends. We would be like one big happy family. What could possibly go wrong? Turns out that teenage drama, hormones, and angst had other plans. While we still remain friends to this day, we have all gone our own separate ways in regard to relationships.

These images and plans stayed with me as I grew older. In college, I started to add the fantasy wedding to the mix. I almost ended up scaring away my then boyfriend (who eventually became my husband) because I was looking through wedding magazines after we had only been dating for a couple of months. He even asked me if I really liked him for who he was or if I liked him because he fit the mold of the husband I wanted in my fantasy wedding! (I have to admit, he did bear a slight resemblance to the man from my old JC Penney catalogs!)

My immediate answer was an emphatic "No!" but his question did make me stop to think about my true feelings. I had to do some real soul searching to make sure I wasn't simply trying to fit another piece of my dream life puzzle into place. I am so glad I did because it turns out that while my husband isn't the man from the catalog (I've never seen him rock a high top fade), he is the perfect man for me.

To quote an adapted line from Robert Burns' poem, "To a Mouse," "The best-laid plans of mice and men often go awry." No matter how carefully a project is planned, something may still go wrong with it. As my best-laid plans turned out, I didn't get married at twenty-three. Although I did marry my college boyfriend who I began dating when I was twenty, we did not get married until I was twenty-nine. When we married, we were in a long-distance relationship due to our jobs. That job situation continued for several more months until I was able to secure a transfer to move closer to him. We decided to wait a few years until I was thirty-two to enjoy married life before expanding our family. We were operating under the delusion that with one trip to Mexico we would be pregnant, right? At least that is what a ton of romance novels always boast. Unfortunately, life is not always as predictable as a romance novel or a dream board or a family plan made with a friend.

And so, our journey was just beginning.

Introduction

This book of devotionals is to help those who have struggled and continue to struggle with conception. Infertility is not an easy road with a quick fix that will make everything okay. However, with prayer and meditation on the Bible's promises, you can come out stronger and closer to God (the ultimate Creator). During the next twenty-eight days (the average time-span of a woman's cycle), use this devotional to help you dig deeper when studying the Word of God to increase your hope, faith, and knowledge of God's everlasting love.

WEEK 1
Menstrual Phase: And Another One

The menstrual phase is the first stage of a woman's monthly cycle. It's also when *menses* (or your period) begin. This phase starts when an egg from the previous cycle isn't fertilized. Because pregnancy hasn't taken place, the levels of the hormones estrogen and progesterone drop. The thickened lining of your uterus, which would support a pregnancy, is no longer needed, so it sheds through your vagina. During your period, you release a combination of blood, mucus, and tissue from your uterus.[1]

My introduction to womanhood came on a beautiful winter day. The sun was shining bright, the birds were chirping, and the freshly fallen snow was dressing the ground with a crisp, clean white landscape. Doesn't that depiction sound lovely? In reality, I don't really remember much about the start of my period except it happened shortly after I turned twelve, and I was really uncomfortable. My biological mother had passed away a few years prior to my twelfth birthday, so I was living with my father, stepmother, and two sisters.

My stepmother was a wonderful help during this time except she didn't have the same relationship with "Aunt Flo" that I did. When all of the ladies in our household had eventually started their menstruation cycles, it turns out that I was the only one out of the four of us with whom "Aunt Flo" had an adversarial relationship. My period came like clockwork each month (yay), but it also came with a vengeance (boo). I assumed the extremely heavy cycles I endured would be my lot in life.

I remember my stepmom warning me once, "Oooh, Kelli, you better not ever even think of having sex. With your periods, as soon as someone even kisses you, you'll get pregnant!"

I might have relied a little too much on this word of advice for too long. I thought with the regularity of "Aunt Flo," I had nothing to worry about like my biological mother who had conceived me seven years after her wedding and my younger sister almost four years later. I honestly believed that the first time I had unprotected sexual intercourse I would get pregnant.

In fact, I was banking on it. I really did go on a trip to Mexico thinking, "Five days in the sun, and I'll come home with a bun in the oven." That intention didn't really go as planned... "Aunt Flo" actually came to visit while we were in Mexico. But I was still encouraged... *I will have next month, right?*

Next month became next year, and I soon looked up and realized that we had been trying for almost two years with no luck in sight. By this time, I was close to thirty-five and was starting to get a little nervous. I started searching the Internet and learned that The American Society for Reproductive Medicine recommends that a woman should consult her health-care provider if she is: under thirty-five years old and has been trying to conceive for more than twelve months, or over thirty-five years old and has been trying to conceive for over six months.

I contacted my OB-GYN to obtain a recommendation for a fertility specialist within my insurance network. While waiting for my appointment, I started researching different ways that fertility specialists could help. I convinced myself that I would probably be fine and possibly end up with twins, so this visit and treatment would be a one-shot-and-done win!

In January of 2016 I made an appointment with a fertility specialist to discuss the issues that I had been experiencing. I filled out a standard questionnaire and was surprised when the fertility specialist called me back prior to my first appointment to dig a little deeper into my situation. It turns out that my heavy menstrual flow and lack of conception made him think that I might have *endometriosis*. I pulled the phone away from my ear and stared at it for a beat before asking him to repeat what he had said. You see in all my thirty-five years of life, I had never heard of endometriosis. My appointment was scheduled for the following day, but as soon as we got off the phone, I jumped on the Internet and started doing my own research—again.

According to the Mayo Clinic, *endometriosis* is an often painful disorder in which tissue similar to the tissue that normally lines the inside of a woman's uterus—the *endometrium*—grows outside the uterus. The symptoms of this condition include painful periods, pain with intercourse, pain with bowel movements or urination, excessive bleeding, and infertility. Not until this conversation with my fertility specialist was I ever aware that saturating a super-plus sized tampon and sanitary napkin in an hour to an hour and a half was considered excessive bleeding.

My only frames of reference for menstrual cycles were my stepmom and my sisters. None of them had cycles similar to mine in frequency, duration, or quantity. I simply thought, *I am a typical heavy bleeder. Don't most ladies have to sleep with mattress protectors and towels during that time of the month?* I had never experienced any of the other symptoms the specialist had mentioned—only the exception of the inability to conceive. Even after reading various articles on the subject, I still wasn't dismayed. After all, I was now seeing a fertility specialist, which meant he knew the best ways for me to get pregnant. My family expansion dream would only take a bit longer.

After that first visit with the doctor, I learned that the only true way to determine if a woman has endometriosis is to have a *laparoscopy*, an outpatient surgical procedure. During a laparoscopy procedure, a tiny incision is made near the woman's navel, and a slender viewing instrument (laparoscope) is inserted to look for signs of endometrial tissue outside of the uterus. This relatively painless procedure confirmed the doctor's suspicions, and I was diagnosed with Stage 4 endometriosis. After the laparoscopy procedure, my doctor consulted with my husband and me about the extent of endometrial growth in my uterus, colon, intestines, ovaries, and appendix. Hearing this information was shocking to say the least. My doctor looked at me and asked, "Are you sure you have never felt any pain?"

He then informed us that if I didn't undergo further surgery, I would most likely end up in an emergency room within the next two years due to the shifting of my internal organs from the extensive endometrial growth. *Yikes!*

As scary as the diagnosis was, the next part of the treatment plan was fear-inducing. The extensiveness of the endometrial growth would require my undergoing a much more invasive surgery. In preparation for this surgery, I would have to see several different specialists who would all have a part in "putting me back together" again. I had previously been told that I had a naturally low iron count. I learned the endometriosis could have played a factor in this diagnosis as well. Unfortunately, my low iron count meant that I would need iron infusions to boost my levels high enough to proceed with the surgery.

The week before my surgery was scheduled, my iron levels were tested again. Unfortunately, the infusions had not produced the desired results. My sister and I ended up staying in the hospital for most of that Friday as I was receiving two blood transfusions so that I would be stable enough for the surgery.

The day of the surgery came quickly. I donned the standard hospital garb, signed all the required forms and mentally hyped myself up for the procedure. My husband and younger sister accompanied me. We were told that the procedure would take a few hours, so everyone prepared for the wait. A few hours turned into seven due to the severity of my disease. I cannot imagine what it must have felt like for my family to have to hear the news that the surgery was taking longer than initially expected.

I remember coming into the recovery room and being vaguely aware of what was going on. For some reason, as I was rolled back to my hospital room, my only thoughts involved how I was going to pee. I now know that people say strange things when coming out of anesthesia! My first few days in the hospital were filled with pain and were uncomfortable. The six weeks of recovery after that hospital stay was no walk in the park either. However, I was still optimistic that the pain and time of convalescence was all worth it because soon I would be pregnant.

My husband and I met with the fertility specialist a few weeks after the surgery to discuss the next steps. We were told that due to my low egg count (I mean, come on, folks. I just couldn't catch a break.) and the fact that a portion of my ovaries had to be removed during the surgery, the option with the most potential for success was for us to proceed with in vitro fertilization (IVF).

When I was growing up, fertility challenges were never addressed. I come from a large, VERY fertile family, so there seemed to be no reason for these conversations to take place. Even after hearing the story of Sarah in the Bible, I didn't put two and two together to realize that sometimes women didn't have children—not because they chose not to, but because they couldn't. Suffice it to say, I was incredibly uncomfortable with the idea of IVF when the subject was first proposed. I know that my considerations may seem silly, but in my mind, the thought that kept going through my brain was if I had to go the IVF route, maybe God didn't want me to conceive. I mean, it's not NATURAL, right?

The decision-making process of whether or not to pursue IVF was one of soul searching. When it came down to it, what made us decide to proceed were two Bible verses:

"Every good gift and every perfect gift is from above, and cometh down from the father of lights, with whom is no variableness, neither shadow of turning." – James 1:17 (KJV)

"And God blessed them, and God said unto them, Be fruitful, and multiply, and replenish the earth." – Genesis 1:28a (KJV).

God has given us all gifts and talents uniquely chosen for each individual in order to accomplish His will on this earth. It not only takes practice to be a doctor, but it can also be a gift for those who use their skills to better the world. Our doctor was not only highly skilled, but I believe that he was operating in the gift that God had blessed him with to help others "be fruitful" in the area of conception. Our decision was made based on these considerations.

A few months later, after healing from the surgery, a crazy amount of doctor appointments and hormone injections (ouch), the day came for us to check to see how many eggs were ready for extraction. The fall day that had started out with so much promise ended with heartache. I didn't have enough eggs that were the right size to continue with the procedure. Devastation swamped me. Seemingly every time I thought we were moving closer to our goal, something in my body actively worked against it. I cried, and I asked God, "Why?" But my spirit wouldn't let me stop there. In order to start healing, I had to start moving out of my anger and hurt.

Looking back on this time of my life, I know now that I needed to let myself grieve for the loss of this dream. I tend to internalize many of my feelings, always trying to be the strong one, but I want you to know that being sad is okay. Working through your grief is essential for healing, but you must work THROUGH it. Don't wallow in despair because God still has plans for you.

In 2 Samuel 12:15-24, the Bible shares King David's grief regarding the death of his and Bathsheba's first child. If David had continued to wallow in his grief for his child, he would have missed the opportunity to be a comfort to his wife. My husband also needed support during this time of despair for us. Had David continued to grieve, he may have missed the blessing of conceiving another child.

Life continued to move on. After about six months, my husband and I discussed trying one more round of IVF, which is an incredibly expensive process. Fortunately for us, my husband's insurance coverage was enough for two rounds of treatment. Almost a year to the date of our first effort, I received a phone call from my doctor letting me know that all three—THREE—of our viable eggs were successfully inseminated! We were so excited!! We only had to wait a few more days to see which ones made it to the "Day 5" stage and became embryos.

I was so happy to see the doctor's office phone number show up on my phone later that week. Unfortunately, we didn't receive happy news this time. He relayed the news that none of the eggs were viable for transfer. We couldn't believe it. *This cannot be happening again.* Not only did the procedure not work, but we were also informed that my egg count reserves were now so low that the possibility of having a future successful IVF was almost non-existent. Our best option at this point would be to use "donor eggs."

This news was harder to take than before because not only had I felt like I had lost three actual children (I mean sperm met egg and got happy), but I felt like a failure as a woman because there was almost no chance that my eggs would ever be enough to create a child with my husband. I was sad, hurt, ashamed, and most importantly angry. "Aunt Flo" had lied!

---

1. Stephanie Watson, "Stages of the Menstrual Cycle," Healthline, last modified March 29, 2019,
https://www.healthline.com/health/womens-health/stages-of-menstrual-cycle#menstrual.

DAY 1
You Better Hustle

Devotional Reading:
Genesis 1

Key Verse:
"And God blessed them, and God said unto them, Be fruitful, and multiply, and replenish the earth, and subdue it: and have dominion over the fish of the sea, and over the fowl of the air, and over every living thing that moveth upon the earth."
– Genesis 1:28

Keyword Definition:
Hustle — busy movement and activity

Growing up in Detroit, you either learned how to hustle (line dance) at an early age, or you learned how to act like you knew how to do it! From weddings to barbeques to day parties, once a song like Stevie Wonder's "My Eyes" begins playing, everyone shoots to their feet to groove to the beat. One of the most recognized hustle dances is the "Cha-Cha Slide" by Mr. C the Slide Man. In this hustle dance song, Mr. C regularly calls out specific dance instructions that the participants have to follow in order to keep up with the music and not end up turned in the wrong direction (oh, the horror!). While following the instructions may seem like an easy task, if you're not listening carefully to everything Mr. C is saying, you could easily run into someone, slide right instead of left, and crisscross when you should be reversing. The result? Good-natured boos tell you to get off the dance floor!

Just like a dancer's reputation rests on his ability to listen, understand and follow the directions of the DJ when dancing to a hustle, it's important for us to follow the specific commands that God has given us to fulfill the plans that He has for us. The Bible serves as our handbook to help us know the desires of God. The very first edict given to man, which is given in the first chapter of the first book of the Bible, is to be fruitful, multiply, replenish, subdue and have dominion over the earth.

What is God really asking us to do? Let's look at the definition of each word for understanding.

1. *Fruitful* — "To bear fruit, to increase, to grow." What type of fruit (Galatians 5:22, 23) are you producing in your life? Since we know that people are influenced not only by their DNA, but also by the environment in which they grow up, what characteristics will you be passing onto your future children?

2. *Multiply* — "To become great, to become many, to enlarge." While you are "in your meantime" period, in what ways are you enlarging your territory of influence to draw others to Christ?

3. *Replenish* — "To be filled, satisfied, accomplished." Are you seeking the contentment that only God can provide for your current situation?

4. *Subdue* — "To bring into bondage." Are you asking the Holy Spirit to help you bring all negative thoughts about your current situation into captivity so that

peace can reign in your spirit?

5. *Have Dominion* — "To rule, dominate." Are you stepping into the leadership role calling for you? Are you being a support system for your spouse who is sharing this journey with you?

Fulfilling this command may seem like an overwhelming responsibility, but God knows our strengths, weaknesses, and limitations. More importantly, He knows how to pull the best out of us because He is our Creator. I know as a woman trying to conceive reading that Scripture can sometimes be hard. I can feel like I failed in the very first instruction God gave me—like I'm stomping instead of hopping... and offbeat at that! But even though today may be the start of another visit from "Aunt Flo," please don't be discouraged. Just like the DJ's call and response will repeat, God will bless you with another chance to accomplish His directive.

Things to Ponder...

1. What are some ways that you can be fruitful during this time?

2. Are you replenishing your spirit with the Word of God?

3. Over what is God specifically calling you to have dominion? In today's reading, He tells us to *rule over*, i.e., be responsible for the welfare of all His creations on earth. That's a large task for a single person to fulfill, but you can find one or two ways that you can make a significant impact.

Scriptures for Inspiration

Exodus 1:7, Leviticus 26:9, Psalm 105:24

DAY 2

God's Creative Power: No Assistance Required

Devotional Reading:
Genesis 2

Key Verse:
"And every plant of the field before it was in the earth, and every herb of the field before it grew: for the LORD God had not caused it to rain upon the earth, and there was not a man to till the ground." – Genesis 2:5

Keyword Definition:
Till — prepare and cultivate the land for crops

Let's talk about God's power as displayed in His creations. We know from Genesis 1 that God created all plants, birds, animals, fish, insects, bodies of water, lands, and celestial bodies through the power of a single phrase: "Let there be...." It's easy to read over these words quickly without giving any real thought to their significance. To help us gain a better perspective of the true magnificence of God's creative power, I want to look at one aspect—the birds—of His opus in four dimensions.

A *dimension* is defined as "a measurable extent of some kind." Every physical thing in this world can be described in terms of dimensions. As a quick reminder, the first four dimensions are length, height, depth, and time. The first three dimensions build upon each other. For example, if you are explaining something in the second dimension, you are expressing both its length and height.

Dimension 1: Length. Typically, length is expressed as a measurement in a straight line. In terms of reading God's Word, it is like reading without putting anything into context.

Dimension 2: Height. This dimension is like looking at a picture of a bird drawn on a flat piece of paper. You can see its shape but haven't yet understood the full complexity of the fowl. For reading the Bible, you are doing more than simply reciting the words; you are also gaining comprehension.

Dimension 3: Depth. The bird can now be viewed from all angles. At this point, you are not only reciting and comprehending God's Word, you are also applying it to your life.

Dimension 4: Time. The bird is now seen in movement. The testimony of your application of God's Word in your life can now serve to encourage others.

Did you know that recent research by the American Museum of Natural History found that there are over 18,000 different species of birds? This number doesn't even take into account all the varieties of colors and speckles that each individual bird may have. If God has this much power and precision when it comes to fashioning each bird, what makes you think He is not even more particular about the creations He made in His own image?

In today's reading God reminds us not only of His power over creation, but also His power to sustain and encourage us to grow—without any assistance needed. God has the ultimate power to override any obstacle conception struggles have put before Him. Nothing is too hard or impossible for God. He did not need Adam's help to till the ground for the vegetation in the garden of Eden to grow. He doesn't need our help in reversing barrenness from our womb. He only asks for our faith, trust, and obedience in following His will. Thank God that we are not in this journey alone.

Things to Ponder...

Think of one thing that God created that has left you in awe.

1. How unique is this creation?
2. How has God protected and provided for it?
3. What inspiration can you derive from God's attention in this creation?

Scriptures for Inspiration

Matthew 6:25-34

DAY 3
Check the Receipts!

Devotional Reading:
Genesis 3

Key Verse:
"And when the woman saw that the tree was good for food, and that it was pleasant to the eyes, and a tree to be desired to make one wise, she took of the fruit thereof, and did eat, and gave also unto her husband with her; and he did eat."
– Genesis 3:6

Keyword Definition:
Hearsay — information received from other people that one cannot adequately substantiate; rumor

Have you noticed that when you're trying to eat healthy and shopping for non-perishable (boxed, canned, bagged) items, you tend to gravitate toward items that have predominantly green packaging or lettering? Did you know that the color of a food's packaging actually invokes thoughts and/or emotions to help us determine what we buy? Multiple studies have been conducted on the psychology of food packaging color, and the subject is amazing. Consider the following determinations:

- Black items tend to represent luxury and authority (organic snacks, protein shakes).
- Red items bring forth thoughts of passion, boldness, and appetite (peanut butter, chips).
- Green makes you think of growth, nature, health (low-fat frozen meals; alternative protein sources).
- Blue evokes thoughts of trust and reliability (nicely boxed pasta).

But while the color of the packaging might seduce you into choosing a particular type of cookie, if you aren't careful about reading the ingredients list, you may be deceived into getting more or less than what you've paid for. For example, that healthy cookie may be lower in calories but chock full of unnatural preservatives and flavorings to make up for the calorie deficit.

Today's story is a perfect example of getting deceived by the packaging, or in other words, folks not taking the time to check the ingredients list (or as young people say, "Check the receipts.") I'm relatively sure we've all heard the story of how the serpent tempted Eve with the fruit, and after falling victim to his lies, she passed on the fruit to Adam to take a bite. While the story may seem simplistic in nature, digging a little deeper will help in understanding the things we should be checking when seeking recommendations from others regarding our conception options.

1. **It's not enough to *know* better; you have to *do* better.** Eve knew God's specific command in regard to the fruit of that one tree (vv. 2, 3). When questioned about it, she could cite letter and verse of what God had dictated. Yet she was able to be swayed against her own better judgment. We can easily look at Eve and

think we would have made a different choice, but when faced with alternatives to God's instructions, haven't we fallen short (sinned)? The reason why Bible study is so important is because it helps you internalize what God is speaking to you. It lets you learn His voice. But God is also asking us to take the knowledge that we internalize from our study and prayer and apply it to our everyday situations. Employ it to when you're seeking out which OB-GYN or fertility specialist to see. Implement His truths in determining which adoption path you want to take. Don't simply *know* the Word; *use* the Word to help you make decisions in life.

2. **The more you "hear" God's voice, the better you'll be able to distinguish His from other voices.** While Eve definitely knew God wasn't speaking to her in the physical sense (vv. 4, 5), she let her own desire to be more knowledgeable and perhaps even closer to God distort her ability to discern that the serpent wasn't speaking to her for her good. How can her desire to be more knowledgeable and closer to God be bad? I think the desire itself isn't the issue but her method to obtain the closeness. She was looking at the serpent's suggestion as a shortcut to God instead of putting in the time and effort to continue to build her relationship with Him. Part of developing that relationship with God instead of "microwaving" it is that your ability to recognize truth grows. Are you pursuing God's voice when you seek advice from other people in regard to your situation to help you determine what's valid and what's false? Many people have been swayed by false promises given with good intention.

The following are a few examples of some false old wives' tales or hearsay that people have followed for years regarding conception:

a. Certain intercourse positions matter when trying to conceive.

   b. If you start trying to adopt, then you'll conceive.

   c. Wearing rose quartz increases fertility.

   d. You can't get pregnant while breastfeeding.

   e. Exercise negatively affects your fertility.

3. **What's good for the goose isn't necessarily good for the gander.** The whole issue I have with Adam here, and yes, I have an issue with Adam, is that everyone always blames Eve for our misfortunes in getting kicked out of Eden, but hardly ever look to Adam's role. Now I'm not saying that you shouldn't trust that the food that your spouse gives you isn't good for you, but think about it like this:

   a. If God gave Adam the responsibility of tending to everything in the garden of Eden (Genesis 2:15), why didn't he recognize the fruit he was given as coming from the tree of the knowledge of good and evil? My assumption is that God would make the fruit of that tree look different from every other tree. After all, why would God try to trick His children into sinning?

   b. Instead of taking responsibility for his own actions, Adam quickly tried to shift the blame to Eve (v. 12). Notice that they didn't feel ashamed of what they had done until they heard God's voice in their midst. Instead of taking time out to repent for the sin of eating of this tree upon immediately recognizing his error (whether or not it was a sin of omission), Adam and Eve started making themselves clothes to hide their shame (v. 7).

The takeaway from these considerations is that simply because Eve was seemingly enjoying the fruit didn't mean that Adam had to try it out too. The advice, treatment, retreat for one person in order to get pregnant may not necessarily work for you. Don't blindly follow after the newest craze simply because it looks appealing. Once again, stop to pray and then listen to what God is telling you. He's always speaking; we just have to be willing to listen. For additional practical applications, the following are some great tips when seeking out an OB-GYN, a fertility specialist, or an adoption agency.

OB-GYN Tips[3]	Fertility Specialist Tips[2]	Adoption Agency Tips[1]
If you have any high-risk issues, make sure the doctor has experience in this situation.	Do some research.	Find one where you feel you're heard and supported.
Make sure they are board-certified.	Trust your instincts (Holy Spirit Nudge).	Ensure good ethical commitment and quality counseling services.
Be honest with your doctor about your history and your family's health history.	Don't choose solely based on insurance coverage.	Make sure you feel free from coercion or pressure.
Make sure you feel comfortable... this is an intimate relationship and awkwardness need not apply.	Be wary about non-transparent results on their websites.	Make sure they clearly communicate your rights.
If you guys work well together, stay with them.	Find out how many IUI, IVF procedures they normally do.	The agency should respect and honor the commitments to both the expectant parents and the birth mother/father.
	How experienced/well trained are the doctors?	
	What are you getting for your money?	
	Seek out support groups.	

Things to Ponder...

1. Can you think of anything that you may have been "tricked" into trying in your effort to conceive that could have been prevented with a quick check from the Holy Spirit?

2. What are ways that you can help to develop your "ear" skills in order to know what God's voice sounds like?

Scriptures for Inspiration
2 Timothy 2:15, 1 John 4:1, 1 Kings 3:9

---

1. "Choosing an Adoption Agency," National Council for Adoption, published 2014, http://www.adoptioncouncil.org/ expectant-parents/find-an-agency.

2. Ruben Castaneda, "How to Find a Good Fertility Clinic," U.S. News and World Report, April 30, 2018, https://health.usnews.com/health-care/patient-advice/articles/2018-04-30/how-to-find-a-good-fertility-clinic.

3. Elaine K. Howley, "How Can I Find the Best OB-GYN?" U.S. News and World Report, March 26, 2018, https://health.usnews.com/health-care/patient-advice/articles/how-can-i-find-the-best-ob-gyn.

DAY 4
A Dormant Branch

Devotional Reading:
Genesis 11:10-32

Key Verse:
"But Sarai was barren; she had no child." – Genesis 11:30

Key Word Definition:
Barren — incapable of producing offspring; devoid, lacking

Have you ever noticed a tree whose branches look sickly? The limbs are bare, and the leaves are shriveled or missing. You might think that the tree is dead and needs to be removed, cut down and/or replaced with a more "lively" one. Before you get out the chainsaw to cut it down, STOP and take a minute to check to see if it's only in a dormant state.

As per the SFGate website, "Dormant branches are simply resting temporarily before they spring to life again, while dead branches cannot revive themselves. A dead branch and a dormant branch may look similar from a distance, but up close each exhibits subtle characteristics that define its state of life."[1]

To the outsider looking in, Sarai, a married woman of some years, was perceived to be like a dead tree limb. By not providing her husband with children, at that time, she was looked down upon. If that wasn't enough, the proceeding verses in chapter eleven seem to flaunt the fact that everyone (her sisters-in-law included) was getting pregnant but her.

"Now these are the generations of Terah: Terah begat Abram, Nahor, and Haran; and Haran begat Lot. And Haran died before his father Terah in the land of his nativity, in Ur of the Chaldees. And Abram and Nahor took them wives: the name of Abram's wife was Sarai; and the name of Nahor's wife, Milcah, the daughter of Haran, the father of Milcah, and the father of Iscah." – Genesis 11:27-29 (KJV)

But God had a different plan. While we first read about Sarai's "barrenness" in chapter eleven of Genesis, later in this same book we can look forward to her "fruitfulness" in chapter twenty-one. Sarai's womb wasn't dead; it was just in a dormant state waiting for instructions from God to end its "temporary rest and spring to life."

Things to Ponder

1. What area of your life is going through a dormant phase right now?

2. How do you react to hearing about other people receiving the blessings of pregnancy while you're still in your dormant stage?

3. Why do you think it was important for God to "call out" Sarai's condition in this single verse?

4. How are you handling your "meantime"?

Scripture for Inspiration
Psalm 113:9

1. Victoria Lee Blackstone, "Difference Between Dead & Dormant Branches," sfGate, accessed August 31, 2020, https://homeguides.sfgate.com/difference-between-dead-dormant-branches-85029. html#:~:text=Dormant%20branches%20are%20simply%20resting,are%20dead%20or%20simply%20dormant.

DAY 5
Seeds and Sand

Devotional Reading:
Genesis 13:12,14-18

Key Verse:
"And I will make thy seed as the dust of the earth: so that if a man can number the dust of the earth, then shall thy seed also be numbered." – Genesis 13:16

Key Word Definition:
Dust — fine, dry powder consisting of tiny particles of earth or waste matter lying on the ground or on surfaces or carried in the air

Have you ever thought about how much dust there is on the earth? Dust can be comprised of many objects, including pollen, bacteria, smoke, ash, salt crystals from the ocean, and small bits of dirt or rock, including sand. From previous devotional readings, it's known that Abram was dwelling in the land of Canaan when God spoke to him. We can assume that his view of the landscape surrounding him was that of a desert. If we simply try to quantify the amount of "sand" dust in Abram's view, it must have been astounding.

To give you a grasp of how far and wide God promised for Abram's descendants to grow in number, think about how many grains of sand in a simple 8-oz cup contains. Since sand particles can range in size, we will assume for our purposes that a typical grain of sand can sit in a 0.5 mm square. Now to do some math:

- 1 liter = 100 mm cube ==> 8 million grains of sand in a 1-liter container.

- 8 oz cup = 250 ml ==> 250 ml = 1/4 liter ==> 2 million grains of sand in an 8 oz cup.

So, stop. Really try to put these measurements into perspective. God told Abram that his "seed would be numbered as the dust of the earth." I don't need to do anymore math to know that the earth contains far more than one or two 8-ounce cups of sand! Can you imagine how Abram must have felt at hearing this promise from God twice? (See Genesis 12:2.) Abram was already 75 years old at this point in his life. While we know that in the early years of the world men often didn't start having children until after their centennial birthday, the majority of the last seven generations of Abram's line had all started having kids when they were much younger. Having children this late in life during Abram's time wasn't unprecedented, but it seemed like fewer and fewer people were waiting so long. One fact never really mentioned in the Bible before Abram and Sarai's story is how old the women were who conceived. At the time of God's initial promise to Abram, Sarai was already sixty-five years old!

While men have an infinite supply of "little swimmers," women are born with a finite number of eggs. With every cycle that we go through during our fertile years, our chances of conception decrease because we have fewer eggs to fertilize. What amazing faith Abram and Sarai had to have not only to be in a position to hear and know God's voice, but also to believe that what He promised would come true! Can you have faith like Abram to look upon all of the sand in your eyesight (to the north, south, east and west) and know that you, who have never fathered a child, would be the patriarch to so many?

The next time you are at the beach or gardening in your yard, grab a handful of sand and/or dirt and praise God. Just like He promised Abram that his "seed shall be numbered like the dust of the earth," He can choose to bless you with the same promise. What He did for one of His faithful servants, He can do for you too, and your seed will be like sand.

Things to Ponder

1. About what is God calling you to have massive faith?
2. Are you limiting God's greatness by forgetting how powerful He is?
3. What would your reaction be in the face of God's promise?
4. Are your ears open to hearing God speak His promises to you?

Scriptures for Inspiration
Hebrews 11:1; Acts 10:34-35

DAY 6
An Appointed Time

Devotional Reading:
Genesis 18:1-16

Key Verse:
"Is there anything too hard for the LORD? At the time appointed I will return unto thee, according to the time of life, and Sarah shall have a son." – Genesis 18:14

Key Word Definition:
Appointed — (of a time or place) decided on beforehand; designated

As I was preparing to write this devotional in March 2020, I flipped through the previous pages of my notebook and found my prayer list from March 2016. When I was writing out that prayer list, I was recovering from having the laparoscopy procedure (to determine if I had endometriosis) and preparing my mind and body for my upcoming myomectomy surgery (to remove said found endometriosis) so that I could increase my chances of getting pregnant. My prayer list from that particular day called out... "get pregnant in 2016 and birth a healthy child".

Looking back on that prayer list four years later, while I can see how some of my prayers have been answered (although not all in the way I was expecting), this specific request was denied (at least for the year 2016). When going through the devotional reading today, I can definitely understand Sarah's frustration and doubt...it was going on the twenty-fifth year since God had made His initial promise to Abraham (Genesis 12:2). At the age of ninety years old, it's easy to want to laugh (or huff, roll your eyes, or say "ooooooooo-kay") when you hear someone say, "You are going to have a child." Maybe Sarah didn't realize it was God talking (our internal doubts can often make it harder to hear God's voice) or maybe she was too consumed with how large her problem seemed, but we must always try to remember how truly BIG our God really is!

Review verse fourteen again. We can see that God had already laid out a specific time frame for a specific thing to happen, not only in Abraham and Sarah's lives, but in our lives also. God carefully and particularly plans out what He wants for us to accomplish/have/achieve in our lives. This is why we are each given different gifts, talents, and passions in order to best accomplish His purpose, but we have to be tuned into Him to know how we are to proceed.

I have hope in God knowing that although four years have gone by since my March 2016 prayer request, as the saying goes, "Delayed does not equal denied." I am putting my trust in God and opening my ears to hear what He wants to tell me about my path to motherhood and every other request in my life.

Things to Ponder

1. What do you do when you feel overwhelmed with doubt?

2. Why did Sarah lie about her doubt (Genesis 18:12, 13, 15)? Why do we lie to God about our doubts?

3. Do you really think that there's nothing too hard for God? What testimony(ies) can you list that demonstrate how BIG God is?

Scriptures for Inspiration
Jeremiah 1:5; 29:11

DAY 7
Forgiveness = Healing

Devotional Reading:
Genesis 20

Key Verses:
"Now therefore restore the man his wife; for he is a prophet, and he shall pray for thee, and thou shalt live: and if thou restore her not, know thou shalt surely die, thou, and all that are thine." – Genesis 20:7

"So Abraham prayed unto God: and God healed Abimelech, and his wife, and his maidservants; and they bare children." – Genesis 20:17

Key Word Definitions:
Infertility — a disease of the reproductive system defined by the failure to achieve a clinical pregnancy after twelve months or more of regular unprotected sexual intercourse (World Health Organization)

Heal — cause (a wound, injury or person) to become sound or healthy again; alleviate (a person's distress or anguish); correct or put right (an undesirable situation).

Restore — bring back (a previous right, practice, custom, or situation); reinstate; return (someone or something) to a former condition, place, or position

Day 7 and Day 8 devotionals are dedicated to the story of Abraham and Sarah's interaction with King Abimelech. The devotional reading of the day tells the story of how one person's fear, instead of faith, started a chain reaction that could have resulted in a death. I tell you, when you really start getting into the Bible, you find so many compelling and high-drama scenarios that you wonder why fiction books even need to exist! I'm not denouncing fiction works because I do love a good space opera or a rom-com, but I am simply pointing out how riveting the Word of God really is.

Once again Abraham fears that because of Sarah's beauty, the king would kill him as her husband so that he could take her as his wife. For all my Bible readers out there, I know you're thinking, *didn't we just read about the* EXACT *same situation happening previously in Genesis 12:9-19?* Why, yes...yes, we did. You would think that Abraham would have learned his lesson that telling a lie, even if it's really only a half-truth, is still wrong and can have devastating consequences. But be honest, how many of us have committed the same sin over and over, yet we still seem to expect a different result?

God comes to King Abimelech in a dream to warn him not to sleep with Sarah because she was truly Abraham's wife. God tells King Abimelech that if he restores an undefiled Sarah to her husband, Abraham will pray for him and he will "live." King Abimelech immediately recognizes God's authority and returns Sarah to Abraham. While most of us would have been fighting mad when confronting Abraham with his treachery, King Abimelech takes a slightly different approach.

1. **God called for Sarah to be restored.** While the focus

of King Abimelech's frustration is with Abraham, Sarah was also partly in the wrong. She went along with her husband's deceit. Why was Sarah not confronted with her part? Because of King Abimelech's decision to obey God's decree to the letter of the law. He restored her by not only returning her to Abraham, but also by gifting Abraham with livestock, servants, money and the freedom to dwell in his land. Even though he had taken Sarah not knowing she was a married woman, he paid restitution to Abraham as if he had been the wronged party.

2. **God tells Abimelech that Abraham will pray for him.** I believe the promise of a prayer from a divine prophet for "life" helped to douse the embers of anger in King Abimelech. At the time of the pronouncement of the prayer in this passage, King Abimelech did not know whether or not the prayer would be for something specific. As previously stated, he did know enough about God's authority to know that if God ordained whatever the prayer was for, it was going to be powerfully awesome.

How do you react when confronting someone who has done you wrong? Are you holding on to bitterness and anger when God has told you not only to forgive but also to restore? Do you know that the lack of forgiveness can result in death not only to you but also to your lineage? Are you blocking your blessing by being disobedient?

Let's take a look at the correlation between the lack of forgiveness and infertility.

Lack of forgiveness — Chronic anger puts you into a fight-or-flight mode, which results in numerous changes in heart rate, blood pressure, and immune response. Those changes, then, increase the risk of depression, heart disease and diabetes, among other conditions.[1]

Stress — Several recent studies have found links between the women's levels of day-to-day stress and lowered chances of pregnancy. For example, women whose saliva had high levels of alpha-amylase, an enzyme that marks stress, took 29 % longer to get pregnant compared to those who had less.[2]

We can summarize this to say that unforgiveness can increase stress in our lives, which in turn can negatively affect our chances of conception. Forgiveness (Genesis 20:7), however, will decrease stress and promote healing (James 5:16) and if in His will, conception (Genesis 20:17).

Things to Ponder

1. Why did Abraham repeat the same sin again in regard to telling who Sarah really was?

2. King Abimelech gave gifts to Abraham after Sarah was returned. Do you ever find yourself going above and beyond the normal when you forgive someone?

3. Everyone's fertility challenges may not be the result of a lack of forgiveness. Regardless, in our ongoing efforts to be closer to God, we must learn to get rid of anything that is hindering that relationship, and that includes not forgiving. Write down any names of people that you need to forgive and ask God to reveal to you if the time has come to go above and beyond.

Scripture for Inspiration
James 5:16

1. "Forgiveness: Your Health Depends on It," John Hopkins Medicine, accessed August 31, 2020, https://www.hopkinsmedicine.org/health/wellness-and-prevention/forgiveness-your-health-depends-on-it.

2. Hallie Levine, "How Stress Can Hurt Your Chances of Having a Baby," Grow by Web MD, accessed August 31, 2020, https://www.webmd.com/baby/features/infertility-stress#

1.

WEEK 2

Follicular Phase: Building Hope

The follicular phase, which overlaps with the menstrual phase, starts on the first day of your period and ends when you ovulate. It starts when the hypothalamus sends a signal to your pituitary gland to release follicle-stimulating hormone (FSH). This hormone stimulates your ovaries to produce around five to twenty small sacs called follicles. Each follicle contains an immature egg. Only the healthiest egg will eventually mature, though on rare occasions, a woman may have two eggs mature. The rest of the follicles will be reabsorbed into your body. The maturing follicle sets off a surge in estrogen that thickens the lining of your uterus, which creates a nutrient-rich environment for an embryo to grow.[1]

I'm a huge fan of quirky crime-solving shows such as *Monk*, *Psych*, or *Bones* because you know at the end of an episode, you've watched someone oddly brilliant solve a seemingly impossible problem in under an hour. Recently, I was watching an episode of *Monk* where the friend of the lead character Monk had vacuumed his living room rug. Monk began to vacuum anew, and as his friend watched, he became increasingly frustrated to see Monk redoing his work! Monk points out, "You went on a diagonal; I like it on a grid." If you know anything about the program, you know that this is typical Monk. Due to his many phobias, Monk exerts his control over as much as he can so he can best manage his life.

During your journey to parenthood, how often have you found yourself trying to compensate for not having control over your fertility by exerting EXTRA control over other aspects of your life? You've downloaded menstruation cycle apps, bought ovulation prediction kits, joined every Facebook support group, read every book, adjusted your diet, increased your exercise time, decreased your stress (while stressing yourself out to decrease it) and yet there is still no change in your circumstance. Hundreds or thousands of dollars have been spent on gadgets, gizmos and endless doctor visits, and it all boils down to even though you've done your best to try to control the situation, creation still is ultimately in God's hands.

Size and weight can be another area of control anxiety for some people. For me, I feel like I've been struggling with my weight since my college graduation. I remember going into Jenny Craig a few weeks after I started working fulltime and thinking, *now I can get back on track.* Unfortunately for me, Jenny Craig was too expensive for my new budget, and I didn't really care for their food selections. My money was wasted and my weight continued to creep up due to my poor eating habits and my lack of exercise. However, I wasn't too discouraged because I was young and knew I still had time to get myself together.

Fast forward fourteen years later and not only was I now thirty pounds heavier, but I was also being told that I have a condition that could be causing me to have difficulty getting pregnant. Like many others, when faced with a situation out of my control, I try to find a way to regain that control. As I have already mentioned, I started researching the causes of endometriosis and possible ways to reduce the recurring buildup of the disease. Trust me, no one wants to have *that* surgery more than once!

Endometriosis feeds off of higher levels of the hormone estrogen. To reduce my estrogen levels, I was recommended to try hormonal birth control pills (not really what I was aiming for), exercise regularly to help lower body fat percentage, avoid large amounts of alcohol (no problem here), stay away from inflammatory foods, and avoid a lot of caffeine (a big struggle for me since I love Coca-Cola Classic). But I figured, hey, this is only the wake-up call that I needed to really get my body in shape to prepare it for conception.

I started exercising regularly (even participated in a 10K run), modified my diet to limit my intake of foods that would boost my estrogen levels, and cut back on my pop intake. While my body was physically starting to look better, my pregnancy test results were still coming back negative every month. I started to spiral back into bad habits because I thought, *why keep pushing myself to be healthy if it isn't changing the outcome?* I was so focused on my physical health that I had neglected the most important part of triumphing over any obstacle—making sure my spiritual health was in order. Like Monk's friend who kept shouting that the rug was clean (i.e., myself at the limits of my abilities, I had not yet gotten the memo that it was time to turn it over to a higher authority and start "vacuuming" in a different direction).

Don't lose hope. In this phase of your journey, I want to encourage you to make your health a priority (exercise more, get fresh air, get good sleep, fuel your body with good foods) in preparation for your future parenthood (whether that's through natural conception, adoption, and/or some other path). But most importantly, strengthen your spirit by drawing closer to God. Just like your body is releasing the follicular stimulating hormone (FSH) to encourage your ovaries to produce eggs, release the power of the Holy Spirit within you to help encourage you to produce good fruits.

---

1. Stephanie Watson, "Stages of the Menstrual Cycle," healthline, updated March 29, 2019, https://www.healthline.com/health/womens-health/stages-of-menstrual-cycle#follicular.

DAY 8

God's Authoritative Power: Open and Close

Devotional Reading:
Genesis 20

Key Verses:
"So Abraham prayed unto God: and God healed Abimelech, and his wife, and his maidservants; and they bare children."
– Genesis 20:17

"For the Lord has fast closed up all of the wombs of the house of Abimelech, because of Sarah Abraham's wife." – Genesis 20:18

Key Word Definition:

Power — the capacity or ability to direct or influence the behavior of others of the course of events

In late 2019 and early 2020, the world was rocked by the discovery and fast spreading nature of coronavirus, COVID-19. In a matter of months, life across the world slowed down, and in some cases, came to an abrupt halt as governments ordered citizens to "shelter in place" and stop all but nonessential work. Economies tanked, thousands died and millions of children were forced to stop attending school all because of a virus roughly a nanometer in size—WAAAAAY smaller than a grain of sand, yet this invisible, odor-free, tricky little bugger had the power to cripple the world almost instantly.

That's what COVID-19 has—power. But do you know who is even more powerful than the current coronavirus? God. Matthew 28:18 says, "Then Jesus came to them and said all authority in heaven and on earth has been given to me." God is all powerful and can do any and everything "above and beyond all that we can ask or think." So, the real question is are we asking AND truly believing that God has this power?

In the conclusion of the Abraham, Sarah, and King Abimelech saga, it tells that King Abimelech's house was experiencing a period of infertility. Today's key verse reveals that the source of the barrenness was at the command of God. Why do you think God chose to close up the wombs in King Abimelech's household? After taking some time to ponder this question, I came up with two possible answers.

1. **So that no one would ever question that Abraham was really the father of Isaac.** The private lives of royalty have never been absolutely private. The news reports oftentimes exaggerate each and everything that the royals of Great Britain do—even the smallest of things are sensationalized to the point where you can't even find where the kernel of truth begins. I recently read an article where the Duchess of Sussex Meghan Markle's former co-star admitted to being propositioned with $70,000 to lie about having a relationship with her. Now while the Internet and tabloids weren't around during the time of Abraham and Sarah, gossip was still alive and well. With King Abimelech's "taking" Sarah (v. 2), even though he "had not come near

her" (v. 4), if there hadn't been a time of barrenness in his household, gossips might have tried to pawn off the king as Isaac's dad. How would that potentiality have affected the people's attitudes toward God's promise?

2. **Just to be able to show us again that God is awesome in His power alone.** God not only caused the wombs of the entire household to close, He OPENED THEM BACK UP! That's true power.

Regardless of what seems like it's being blocked, denied, or closed in your life, remember that you serve an amazing God who has the power to rotor-rooter, approve and open any and everything. Don't let fear over COVID-19, negative news from the doctor's office or adoption agency, or just crazy things at work cause you to minimize God's power. "Don't tell God how big your storm is, tell your storm how big God is." – Unknown

Things to Ponder...

1. What worry are you making bigger than God in your life? Why?

2. Is there anything in your life to which you think God has closed the door? If so, why?

3. We can assume that up until Abraham and Sarah's visit, King Abimelech didn't have kids. Something really interesting to note is that the name *Abimelech* means "father of the king." Isn't it cool to think that all these events happened according to divine will so that even Abimelech's name would be fulfilled? What does your name mean? What destiny could you be walking into?

Scriptures for Inspiration

1 Chronicles 29:11; Matthew 19:26; 1 Corinthians 6:14; Ephesians 3:20

DAY 9
Wait Patiently

Devotional Reading:
Genesis 21:1-7

Key Verses:
"And the LORD visited Sarah as he had said, and the LORD did unto Sarah as he had spoken. For Sarah conceived, and bare Abraham a son in his old age, at the set time of which God has spoken to him." – Genesis 21:1, 2

Key Word Definitions
Patience — the capacity to accept or tolerate delay, trouble, or suffering without getting angry or upset
Experience — an event or occurrence that leaves an impression on someone
Hope — a feeling of expectation and desire for a certain thing to happen; a feeling of trust

When my youngest niece was two years old, I introduced her to the concept of waiting patiently. I know it sounds crazy, but every time she would start to fuss for whatever drama a two year old could be currently enduring, I would look at her, and in a firm voice, say, "Wait patiently." Now, my directive didn't have an immediate effect on her right away but saying it enough times produced the desired result I was seeking. As she started to get a little older, her speech skills increased, and I would have her repeat after me, "Wait patiently" when she would become too impatient. Since this interaction became an almost daily occurrence, soon all I would have to do was say "Wait..." and she would chime in with "patiently."

Kids are so amazing during this time of life. They are like little sponges soaking up every new experience, saying, and feeling they observe. I remember getting a call from my sister a year or so after the "wait-patiently" lessons had begun that still tickles me to this day. My sister had me on Bluetooth speaker while she was driving and had gotten frustrated with a fellow motorist. As she began to raise her voice at the other driver to move, I could hear the sweet voice of my then three-year-old niece in the background saying, "Mommy, wait patiently." The lesson of patience, while often long in learning, is truly worth the reward.

God had made an amazing, incredible, unbelievable promise to Abraham and Sarah that in their golden years they would have a son. What wasn't initially stated, but what occurred, was that it would take twenty-five years for this promise to be fulfilled. I know many of us have been praying and waiting and getting disappointed month after month when God's Word of promise from Genesis 1:28 hasn't been fulfilled in our lives.

Each time Aunt Flo shows up, the test results come back negative, or we're told we are still far down on the list for adoption, it can seem like the promise God gave to each of us will never come to pass. But stop! Can you imagine how Sarah must have felt all that time seeing everyone else conceive? She must have been frustrated to have a front-row seat to an entire barren household getting blessed with fertility (Genesis 20:17) but STILL, she didn't get pregnant.

I want to encourage each of you not to give up hope. God always fulfills His Word. God is increasing our capacity for patience during this process. Scripture tells us that patience produces experience and experience produces hope. The Greek word for *experience* is *dokime* which means "proof or testing of a thing." Isn't it wonderful to know that the patience that is developing in us through this experience is providing PROOF that God is faithful, ever-present, all-powerful, and full of love toward us? And what are we going to need once we start birthing God's promise into life (whether physical children, adopted children and/or ministries and businesses serving expecting mothers)? PATIENCE! While I haven't personally experienced childbirth, from hearing accounts of close friends and family who have, the process is not always quick and easy. You need **patience** not to snap at your spouse for telling you to "just breathe and push!" You can learn from others' **experiences** that you will make it through labor eventually and **hope** that everything will go smoothly during the delivery. So basically, you need God!

Through Abraham and Sarah's twenty-five-year journey to fulfillment of God's promise, we see how God increased their capacity in all three areas:

1. **Patience** (Genesis 17:19-21). Although Abraham and Sarah tried to rush ahead of God, God still let it be known that the blessing He promised would happen in His own timing.

2. **Experience** (Genesis 18:12-13). Abraham had already learned his lesson about laughing at God's promise. His experiences and constantly evolving relationship with God allowed him to be able to immediately recognize when he was in God's presence and respect the words that God was speaking.

3. **Hope** (Genesis 20:17). Sometimes you can only pray people through things that you yourself have experienced.

When times get tough and you feel down, remember that God always fulfills His promises!

Things to Ponder...

1. Why do you find it so hard to be patient with God?

2. We can see in the birthing of Ishmael that running ahead of God can often cause unpredictable results. Part of the turmoil in the Middle East today is due to the disagreements between the first two descendants of Abraham. Can you think of one thing that you may have done that was out of God's timing or done out of impatience of waiting for an answer from God?

3. How do you know when you're being patient versus when you're standing still because you're afraid of moving forward?

Scriptures for Inspiration
James 1:2-3; Romans 5:3-6

DAY 10
Hearing Aids and Contacts Not Required

Devotional Reading:
Genesis 21:8-22

Key Verses:
"And God heard the voice of the lad; and the angel of God called to Hagar out of heaven, and said unto her, What aileth thee, Hagar? Fear not; for God hath heard the voice of the lad where he is." – Genesis 21:17

"And God opened her eyes, and she saw a well of water; and she went, and filled the bottle with water, and gave the lad drink." – Genesis 21:19

Key Word Definitions:

Heard — to have perceived (become aware or conscious of something) with the ear the sound made by (someone or something); to be aware of, know the existence of

Ear — the organ of hearing and balance in humans and other

vertebrates; an organ sensitive to the sound in other animals; the ability to recognize, appreciate, and reproduce sounds, especially in music or language
Opened — move or adjust so as to leave a space allowing access to view; undo or remove a lid, cover or fastening of (a container, package, etc.) to get access to the contents

Today's Scriptures tell of Hagar's preparing to leave life as she had known it for the previous eighteen-plus years. While it hadn't always been easy (Sarah treated her quite badly after she conceived Ishmael [Genesis 16:6]), she had the comfort of knowing where she fit in, that she and her son were always well fed, and that Abraham loved her son. After Isaac came along, Ishmael's place within Abraham's household was thrown into flux when Sarah demanded that Abraham throw out Hagar and Ishmael. Although heartbroken to lose his son, Abraham was comforted by God in knowing that Ishmael would be provided for (v. 13).

As Hagar and Ishmael journeyed through the wilderness with only some bread and a bottle of water, it was easy to see how they would become weary and despondent. What a terrible situation they faced! They were in an uninhabited (no one around) and inhospitable (harsh and difficult) area with only meager supplies to last with no destination, no direction, and no deliverance in sight. Hagar cried and was so distraught about the predicament she and her son were in that she forced him beneath a bush so that she wouldn't have to see his demise. But wait...they were not alone.

How many times have you been in a wilderness situation without adequate energy or the means to do much to change your outcome, with no friends and/or family to call, and not even a comfortable place to lay your weary head to cry? Oftentimes seeing "Aunt Flo" appear after our hopes have been buoyed can feel like the wilderness of infertility is claiming another victim, and our cries, prayers and pleas have gone unheard yet once again. But wait...just like Hagar and Ishmael, you are not alone.

What's really awesome about today's passage is that it's told through the experience of Hagar. While Hagar was the one who lifted up her voice and wept, God responded to the voice of Ishmael. Even Hagar, whom you would think would have been able to hear Ishmael, didn't notice the cries of her son. I love how God can not only respond to those whose voice is loud, but He hears our small voice and our sniffles in our prayer closets or under our covers or when we hold it all in and only cry out inside. God's ears are sensitive to the sounds of our cries. He has the ability to recognize our individual voices, and He knows exactly how much we can bear.

Not only does God hear every type of cry, prayer, and plea that we may make, He also has the power to make change happen. God can open our eyes, adjust our view and/or remove every obstacle in our way so that we can see the clear path that He has created for us to get out of this wilderness of depression, rejection, self-doubt, hurt, and anger in which we can find ourselves. Notice that Hagar's despair didn't kick in until she was out of water (v. 15) and the first thing she saw when God opened her eyes was a well of water—her newfound hope (v. 19). As believers we know that we have access to the never-ending water source of Jesus Christ. We will never have to be thirsty again because His Word will provide all the nourishment that we will need to get through the next twenty-eight-day cycle and beyond.

I encourage you today to rise up and fill up your "bottle" (your heart, your soul, your spirit) with the water of Jesus so that you will be refreshed and renewed for the journey to come.

Things to Ponder...

1. Have you ever been afraid to let yourself cry when confronting disappointing news—like if you shed a tear, it will make it real?

2. Why do you think that God responded to Ishmael's cries, even though the angel acknowledged that Hagar's despair could be heard as well?

3. Thinking back, have there been times when you felt that God didn't hear your plea, but you really weren't ready to open your eyes to see His response?

Scriptures for Inspiration
John 4:13-14; Joshua 1:9

DAY 11

Having God's Ear

Devotional Reading:
Genesis 25:19-24

Key Verses:
"And Isaac intreated the LORD for his wife, because she was barren: and the LORD was intreated of him, and Rebekah his wife conceived." – Genesis 25:21

"Therefore shall a man leave his father and his mother, and shall cleave unto his wife: and they shall be one flesh."
– Genesis 2:24

Intreated (Entreated) — to beg; to indicate the success of a petition; to ask; to beseech (ask someone urgently and fervently to do something; implore); to supplicate (ask or beg for something earnestly or humbly)[1]

Here's a fun grammar lesson for all. Auto-antonyms are words that can mean their own opposite. Crazy! When thinking about conception and enlarging one's family size, it takes both the husband and wife's participation to get the ball rolling. Going back to the beginning of the Bible, the initial directive toward married couples is the notion of leaving the familiar and "cleaving" toward each other. *Cleave* is one of those unexpected auto-antonyms meaning both "to split/sever" as well as "to stick fast to." When studying Genesis 2:24 through its original language translation, *cleave* is the Hebrew words *dabaq* or *kollao*, meaning "to adhere to" or "to join one's self to."

It's important to go back to the basics of marriage when going through this process of fertility challenges. We can often get overwhelmed with appointments, charts, hormone injections, and finances, but I feel that God gives us a great reminder in Genesis 25 of the importance of "cleaving" to your spouse.

Isaac and Rebekah had been married for nearly twenty years without having children. Since we know that Rebekah was called *barren*, no conception had taken place during this time. I believe that while they waited year after year for their family to grow, they got to know each other intimately—their likes, dislikes, hurts, angers, and frustrations—during this quiet time. The delay to their blessing with each passing year only served to draw them closer to each other, to cause them to cleave to each other, but most importantly to grow deeper in their relationship with God.

Today's passage has three distinct takeaways from the "meantime" period for Isaac and Rebekah.

1. **Isaac pleaded successfully on Rebekah's behalf.** Because of his close relationship with God, Isaac was able to boldly argue his case before God on Rebekah's behalf for children. Just like when his father bargained with God on behalf of his nephew Lot and the citizens of Sodom and Gomorrah (Genesis 18:16-33), Isaac knew that because of his connection with God, his time spent communing and sharing his intimate thoughts and feelings with the Most High, that God would not only hear his plea, but also answer it in the affirmative. He didn't need to have the perfect closing argument filled with eloquent alliteration, but he did

need to come humbly before God with an honest heart. In addition, because Isaac cleaved to Rebekah, he knew that the desire of her heart was to bear his children. He was able to go to God on her behalf not only because of his relationship with God but because of his relationship with his wife.

2. **Rebekah had her own relationship with God.** When God answered Isaac's prayer, Rebekah was plagued with a difficult pregnancy. Not only was she expecting a child at a more seasoned age (imagine how that would feel in the time of no epidurals in a desert), but neither did she have access to an ultrasound to know that the twins she carried were the cause of some of her increased distress. However, because of Rebekah's own relationship with God, she not only knew to call out to Him, but she was also able to distinguish His voice to hear His answer. His response was able to give her some answers to her questions and help to calm her anxiety.

3. **God always fulfills His Word.** God made a covenant with Isaac's father Abraham that through Isaac (and his children), nations shall arise (Genesis 17:21). Because we know that God does not lie, Isaac and Rebekah could always rely on that word—especially during their wait.

Champion for your spouse, keep God at the forefront, and know that if He said it, He will do it!

Things to Ponder...

1. Have you actively prayed with/for your spouse in

regard to your fertility challenges?

2. Is it difficult to fully express your feelings during this time with your spouse? If so, why?

3. Have you shared your feelings of anxiety, fear, shame with them regarding this situation?

4. What are some ways you can approach the topic with your spouse, especially if he feels like it's his body that is letting both of you down?

Scriptures for Inspiration
Matthew 19:6; Ephesians 5:31; James 5:16

---

1. James Orr, Ed., "Cleave," *The International Standard Bible Encyclopedia Online,*(Grand Rapids: Wm. B. Eerdmans Publishing Co., 1939), https://www.internationalstandardbible.com/C/cleave.html.

DAY 12

Drought Resistant

Devotional Reading:
Genesis 26:1-14

Key Verse:
"Sojourn in this land, and I will be with thee, and will bless thee; for unto thee, and unto thy seed, I will give all these countries, and I will perform the oath which I sware unto Abraham thy father." – Genesis 26:3

Key Word Definitions:

Famine — extreme scarcity of food; shortage
Drought — a prolonged period of abnormally low rainfall, leading to a shortage of water

I've lived in both Phoenix and Houston and am always amazed when I see flowers blooming in the heat each summer. With temperatures typically reaching a sweltering 100° to 110° respectively for days on end, I am reminded how careful and thoughtful our Creator is to think of all of the diversity of plant life decorating the earth that can withstand the awesome power of the sun.

For dry, hot climates, God has created an array of beautiful yet resilient plants that are able to flourish in difficult circumstances. This reminds me of the famine that Isaac and Rebekah experienced shortly after the birth of their twins. In today's reading, it's noted that similar to the famine that Abraham experienced, another famine has befallen the land where Isaac and Rebekah are dwelling. Instead of heading to Egypt as Isaac's father had done previously (Genesis 12), God tells Isaac to stay in the land which He swore to Abraham as an inheritance. Oftentimes when living life becomes difficult, whether it be job difficulties, marriage strains or fertility woes, we find ourselves seeking greener pastures to help sustain us (i.e., new job postings, divorce attorneys, or gimmicky practices such as physic hotlines or prayers to fertility gods). But God is not calling us to keep moving, especially not in the wrong direction. God is asking us to trust Him and to be still so that He can bless us right where we are. Our blessing is found in our OBEDIENCE.

During the famine or shortage in your life, I'm asking you to focus on the resistance and not the drought. We can draw a wealth of inspiration from drought-resistant plants such as echinacea or the purple coneflower, a perennial flower that loves the full sun and fertile, well-drained soil. This pest-resistant plant, which is unpalatable to deer and other herbivores, is also widely utilized for medicinal use, immune system support, detoxification, and wound healing. The following are some characteristics that the purple cornflower shares with the spiritually drought-resistant.

- Perennial. It is faithful (2 Corinthians 5:7).

- Loves full sun and fertile soil. It is craving for the SON (Romans 5:5).

- Pest and herbivore resistant. It is protected (Psalm 18:1-2).

- Promotes good health. It brings peace and healing (3 John 1:2).

Isn't it wonderful to know that God can walk with us through a tough time in our lives and if we listen to His voice, we can come out with an increase in our faith, protected, full of peace, healed, and with a deeper, more intimate relationship with Him? The best part of this story is that because of Isaac's obedience, he was able to prosper in land, power, goods, and reputation. He came out of the famine in a much better position than when he entered. Today, God is calling us to slow down, stop, and heed His voice. Don't rush to make decisions without first seeking the advice of the Holy Spirit. Listen to the voice of Jesus to know whether you should stay or go. Your decision could make the difference in how you weather the famine that you are in.

Things to Ponder...

1. How do you cope when experiencing a drought/famine situation? Think about how you reacted to hear that you have a shortage of eggs/sperm/money/access to resources/time in order to enlarge your family.

2. What does it mean to be planted in fertile soil? Why is the soil type important?

3. What are some ways you can demonstrate obedience to God during this time in your life?

4. In what areas are you seeking God to prosper?

Scriptures for Inspiration

Psalm 18:1-2; Romans 5:5; 2 Corinthians 5:7; 3 John 1:2

DAY 13
God's Strategic Power: Cracking Open the Jar

Devotional Reading:
Genesis 29, 30

Key Verses:
"And when the LORD saw that Leah was hated, he opened her womb: but Rachel was barren." – Genesis 29:31

"And God remembered Rachel, and God hearkened to her, and opened her womb." – Genesis 30:22

Key Word Definitions:

Strategic — carefully designed or planned to serve a particular purpose or advantage

Have you ever struggled to open a stubborn jar? For me, the lid of a spaghetti sauce jar always seems to be stuck whenever I'm in a hurry to make dinner. Most of the time, my husband is around to help me out of the jam, but what happens when he's not there? Am I forever stuck waiting for his return to make spaghetti or are there other ways to crack it open that don't require brute strength?

I did a quick Internet search on ways to open difficult lids and found out that while our natural inclination is to simply give it the good he-ho try, there are many other ways to achieve the desired outcome that require us to rely on using strategy—not our own limited strength. These strategies made me think of how we women struggling with conception can often find ourselves trying to use all of our natural resources (pry open the jar with our muscles) and forget that we have a better, more strategic source of power (God) into who we can tap in order to be blessed with a child (crack the lid).

The following chart shows the correlation between the different ways to open a difficult jar and the womb. [1]

How to Open a Stuck Lid	How to Open Up Your Stuck Womb
1. Use Heat. Heating up the lid will cause the metal to expand, thereby loosening it up to make it easier to open.	**Zechariah 13:9** - God can use fire to purify us. Sometimes our wombs may be closed because we are struggling with spiritual issues that are manifesting in the physical. Seek God for clarity about your specific reason for your conception challenges. Although the heat can be painful, it also brings forth beauty out of fire (the impurities in gold are removed through fire).
2. Create Friction. Use something that offers traction and resistance because it will increase the grip on the lid while not causing you to have to use more strength.	**Exodus 9:12** - God can use friction to bring about a crazy miracle. Think about it. If God had not hardened Pharaoh's heart, would the powerful acts performed by Moses demonstrating God's supremacy have been conducted and the release of the Israelites from 400 years of captivity been as awe-inspiring? How often do we look to that story to find encouragement when we ourselves are in situations of bondage?

3. Use Leverage. Use something long, smooth and thin enough to get under the lid of the jar to help break the pressure.	**Ephesians 6:17** - God has given us the sword of the Spirit to use as our leverage in this world. The sword, His Word, can help to increase our faith during this time by reminding us of God's power, love, and steadfastness.
4. Tap It With A Spoon. Tapping the outside edge of the spoon helps to dislodge food that has gotten stuck between the lid of the jar and the jar.	**Ephesians 4:22-24** - God is calling us to dislodge our old selves. Barrenness may be caused because we let our old mindset of doubt stay at the forefront. If you haven't expanded your mind to believe that a miracle can occur, you won't recognize it when it happens. Get rid of your old thinking, old corruptible ways, and embrace a renewed spirit.

Today's key verses tell how God had the power to both open and close the wombs of Leah and Rachel. While previous examples of this power were addressed in the Day 8 reading, I wanted to highlight that power doesn't always have to do with strength or the authority to influence. Power is also about the ability to be strategic. God's choice of when, how, and to whom barrenness is given or revoked is exactly that—His choice. However, we do know that God is a planner and sees everything that has, is, and will happen. If God had not opened the womb of Leah, Judah (the lineage from whom Joseph, Jesus' earthly father, descends) would not have been born in the order and at the specified time needed to accomplish God's will. If God had not opened Rachel's womb, her son Joseph would not have been born to later save his family from famine. Remember that God isn't asking us to use our own strength during this time to make conception possible; rather, He's asking us to let Him have reign in every aspect of our lives so that His strategic plan can be fulfilled.

Things to Ponder...

1. In what ways do you see God being strategic in your journey of conception?

2. Can you think of ways that you have used strategic thinking in order to accomplish your plans?

3. Have you therefore achieved different results by use of strategy?

Scriptures for Inspiration
2 Samuel 22:33; Luke 1:37

---

1. Katherine Martinelli, "In a pickle: How to open a stuck jar," SheKnows, June 28, 2012, https://www.sheknows.com/food-and-recipes/articles/963722/in-a-pickle-how-to-open-a-stuck-jar/.

DAY 14
What's Your Why?

Devotional Reading:
Genesis 29, 30

Key Verses:
"And Leah conceived, and bare a son, and she called his name Reuben: for she said, Surely the LORD hath looked upon my affliction; now therefore my husband will love me."
– Genesis 29:32

"And when Rachel saw that she bare Jacob no children, Rachel envied her sister; and said unto Jacob, Give me children, or else I die." – Genesis 30:1

Key Word Definitions:
Envy — a feeling of discontented or resentful longing aroused by someone else's possessions, qualities, or luck
Motivation — the reason or reasons a person has for acting or behaving in a particular way

My oldest niece is thirteen months older than her sister. When she was almost two, her little sister was crying (for reasons I cannot remember) and garnering all the attention of her mom and grandma. I happened to look over at the older sister and witnessed her climbing down from the couch, gently lying down on the floor and proceeding to act as if she had fallen down and hurt herself. I started to laugh as she "play" cried until her mom and grandma came to comfort her—after putting her sister back in the playpen. She wasn't hurt, and I don't think she even really wanted attention; she just didn't want her sister to have all the attention.

We see a similar situation play out between Leah and Rachel in Genesis 29 and 30. Leah, who had very poor eyesight, must have felt as if she was always living in her sister's shadow. She wasn't as beautiful as Rachel and couldn't contribute to the family financially because she couldn't work as a shepherdess like Rachel. All of her insecurities caused her to participate in the trickery her father proposed and resulted in her marrying a man who did not love her (Genesis 29:18, 25, 30). How awful is it to be in an unequal relationship? God chose to show mercy on Leah, knowing she was despised by her husband and blessed her with children. However, instead of being thankful for the opportunity to be a mother, Leah continued to bear children to win her husband's attention.

Rachel didn't face the issue of a lack of love. She was beautiful, a contributing member of the household, and had a flattering figure (Genesis 29:17). Rachel, however, envied Leah because she was able to give Jacob what she could not—children. Her motives were equally as selfish (and dare I say rather over dramatic) as Leah's. You would think that with all of the blessings that God had bestowed upon her, she would have been content, but Rachel let the sin of envy cause her to act irrationally.

Sitting in judgment on Leah and Rachel's reactions is easy, but how many of us have found ourselves in their situations? Are we trying to conceive because we feel the calling from God to be fruitful and multiply the earth or do we have more selfish motives like envy, replacement for what love is missing from our lives, or simply feeling the pressure that society has placed on women? How many times have you overlooked thanking God for the blessings He's already provided because the answer to one of your requests has been delayed and/or denied?

I know I've found myself in that position many times. I've been blessed beyond measure with a wonderful husband, financial security, a great extended family, good health (or the resources to get healthy), but I've still been envious of others who may not have all those things but have children. Envy is a very destructive emotion that can cause you to sin (say and/or do negative things to others) and hold bitterness in your heart, which could result in anger and even turning away from God. Envy for others' blessings needs to be nipped in the bud at its infancy so it doesn't grow into something that we will truly regret.

Thankfully, we serve a compassionate and caring God who knows the true desires of our hearts. If we diligently seek Him, He'll heal us from whatever is stopping us from conception (or turn our desires into His desires so that we are content with how He chooses to bless us).

Things to Ponder...

1. Have you found yourself envious of others who seem to have no issue with getting pregnant? How have you treated them in your internal (heart) and external actions?

2. Why do you desire to have children? Are you seeking a successful conception/birth because you want to be a mother or because of other reasons?

3. Are you holding onto any bitterness in your heart toward God because you haven't been able to conceive? If so, have you been honest with God about your

feelings and asked Him to heal your heart?

Scriptures for Inspiration
Proverbs 14:30; Hebrews 11:6

WEEK 3
Ovulation Phase: Execution Time!

Rising estrogen levels during the follicular phase trigger your pituitary gland to release luteinizing hormone (LH) to start the process of ovulation. Ovulation occurs when your ovary releases a mature egg. The egg travels down the Fallopian tube toward the uterus to be fertilized by sperm. The ovulation phase is the only time during your menstrual cycle when you can get pregnant. You can tell that you are ovulating by the following symptoms:

- a slight rise in basal body temperature
- a thicker discharge that has the texture of egg whites[1]

A couple of years ago, I set a goal of running a 10K. I joined a local running group for women and partnered with a friend to train for this momentous event. We downloaded a running app to outline our training plan and met two to three times a week to practice. Preparation for the 10K not only included following a running plan, but also extended into learning what shoes worked best for my stride and arch, what gear I felt most comfortable wearing (I am not an earbuds person), and sacrificing my leisure time of chilling on the couch to put in additional time just walking and jogging on my off-training days. Weeks of training turned into months, and soon the day of the race was upon me. My stamina and pace had increased, my waistline had decreased, and I was fairly confident that I would be successful. However, I had still not actually run a full 10K at this point.

A few days before the race, I picked up my participant packet and cool race swag and prepared my outfit. I got to the race a little early to make sure I would have a good place in my grouping. My anxiety was high, my heart was beating fast, and I started to break out in a light sweat as I stood in line with my pace group. The clock ticked down and before I knew it, I was off—execution time! The race was tough and pushed me in ways I didn't think possible, but when it was all said and done, I crossed the finish line beating the goal pace I had set for myself. With prayer and putting my faith into action (getting up and training each week), my goal was accomplished!

During this time in your cycle, you might be feeling like it's now your execution time. You've completed your training (getting healthier, preparing your body, attending endless doctor appointments), have gotten the right gear to set you up for success (a calm, relaxing atmosphere) and are now ready to start your race (Netflix and Chill). Remember, preparation is important, but ultimately, God is in control of the outcome. While I went to run the race after months of preparation, it wasn't me who got me over the finish line; it was God. There were times that I wanted to quit—like seeing the 2-mile marker come into view but knowing I still had 4.2 miles more to go. There were times when I had to slow down because my breathing wasn't steady. There were also times when I just said, "Forget it" and took a break to walk. Through it all, God was with me. Yes, I did my part, just like you've been doing your part through proper diet, exercise, sleep, vitamins, hormone shots, ovulation charts, doctor visits, etc., but in the end, God's grace and strength allowed me to cross the finish line. Oh, and what a rush that was!

Enjoy this time of execution with your spouse and believe that if it is in God's will and timing, a child will be conceived.

"Lo, children are an heritage of the LORD: *and the fruit of the womb is his reward."* – Psalm 127:3

---

1. Stephanie Watson, "Stages of the Menstrual Cycle," healthline, updated March 29, 2019, https://www.healthline.com/health/womens-health/stages-of-menstrual-cycle#follicular.

DAY 15
Joined Together

Devotional Reading:
Genesis 29, 30

Key Verse:
"And Jacob's anger was kindled against Rachel: and he said, Am I in God's stead, who hath withheld from thee the fruit of the womb?" – Genesis 30:2

Key Word Definition:

Kindled — light or set on fire; arouse or inspire and emotion or feeling

Have you ever gone camping before? If so, you probably know that one of the most important rules that most campsites enforce is that you must be sure to completely douse the flames of the campfire before leaving. An unchecked spark can reproduce a flame that if not monitored can result in a horrific, destructive forest fire.

Similarly, anger can be ignited quickly if left unchecked; it can result in hurt feelings, unforgiveable actions, and unfortunately, a destroyed marriage. Studies by the Danish Cancer Society Research Center have revealed that couples who do not have a child after fertility treatments are three times more likely to divorce than those who do. After Rachel's initial outburst and plea for Jacob to "give her children" in Genesis 30:1, we see that Jacob's response was to get angry. Let me stop right here to point out the following:

1. **It's okay to be angry.** You're going through a difficult process, and your frustrations can sometimes erupt as an irrational outburst, but don't let the anger get out of control. Douse the embers before they ignite into something that cannot be stopped.

2. **Remember who is truly in control.** We can sometimes find ourselves blaming our spouses for our fertility circumstances, but remember that God is ultimately in control. We must stop looking to our bodies as failing us and fall back to the lessons that we learned in Genesis 20:18, 29:31, and 30:22. God has the power to open even the most tightly shut wombs—wombs that might have been closed due to our own actions (i.e., STDs, abortions, etc.).

When I first read this Scripture, I imagined a "kindled" fire as one that starts immediately. It doesn't have to be stoked into getting bigger; it simply grows on its own. The beauty of this word picture is that fire, while powerful, has an enemy that can kill it just as quickly—water. Isaiah 44:3 states that God will "pour water on the thirsty land, and streams on the dry ground; I will pour out my Spirit on your offspring, and my blessing on your descendants." In moments of frustration, call on God and He will pour out His Spirit on you. We know that the Holy Spirit not only serves as our advocate before God but also as our *comforter*—one who provides consolation. God's Spirit will bring peace into your life and your relationship if you will allow Him.

I loved how quickly Jacob corrected Rachel. As partners on this journey to parenthood, we have to be able not only to vent our frustrations to our spouses but also correct each other and lift up each other if we start to lose focus on God. As married couples, we are to cleave to each other, especially in times of distress. One of the greatest powers of a praying couple is that they are "two," and the Word of God says that "where two or three gather in my name, there am I with them" (Matthew 18:20). Are you sitting down with your spouse and praying away your frustrations or have you allowed the Enemy to isolate you so that your support structure is weakened? It's not too late to douse that flame.

Things to Ponder...

1. Have you let the stress of your fertility challenges build a wedge between you and your spouse?

2. What are some ways that you can douse the flame of bitterness and resentment that may have ignited throughout this process?

Scriptures for Inspiration

Isaiah 26:3; Proverbs 12:4; John 14:16

DAY 16
The Power of a Praying Mother

Devotional Reading:
Genesis 27:41-45, 30:25-31:3

Key Verse:
"And the LORD said unto Jacob, Return unto the land of thy fathers, and to thy kindred; and I will be with thee." – Genesis 31:3

Key Word Definitions:

Ancestor — a person, typically one more remote than a grandparent, from whom one is descended

Prayer — intercession (the action of intervening on behalf of another), supplication (the action of asking or begging for something earnestly or humbly)

Have you ever heard the song by Dorothy Norwood titled "Somebody Prayed for Me?" The congregation sang this song often in the Baptist church when I was growing up. I'll admit that as a child I didn't tend to pay close attention to the lyrics, but as an adult, especially one who is struggling with conception, the words take on an entirely new meaning.

My mother prayed for me, had me on her mind,
She took the time and prayed for me.
I'm so glad she prayed.
I'm so glad she prayed.
I'm so glad she prayed for me.

I mentioned at the beginning of this book how my mother struggled with conception. Because she died when I was young, I never had the opportunity to talk with her about her challenges. I imagine that she experienced many of the same emotions that I've gone through. I'm sure she was disappointed, hurt, angry, sad, and shamed that what should be a natural progression for a young married couple simply wasn't working out for she and my dad. While I don't know the exact thoughts that were running through her mind during the six years it took for my parents to conceive me, I do know that my mother was a woman of incredible faith in God. I can imagine that once myself and sister were born into this world, she whispered a sweet prayer over us that we would not experience the same fertility struggles that she went through. An amazing attribute about our God is His remembrance of the prayers of our mothers, our fathers, our ancestors, and we continued to be blessed because they prayed for us (Deuteronomy 29:13).

Today's reading goes back to when Jacob was still dwelling at home with Isaac, Rebekah and Esau. Once Esau learned that Jacob had not only taken his birthright but had also tricked him out of the blessing that Isaac was planning to bestow upon him, he became so angry he was plotting to kill Jacob. Rebekah overheard the gossip and immediately sent for Jacob so that she could persuade him to leave and not return until his brother's anger had cooled.

I feel relatively sure that Rebekah didn't mean for Jacob to be gone for the twenty years he lived with Laban's family, but her motherly instinct to protect her son overcame her desire to be with him daily. Rebekah's experiences with witnessing that God always answered prayers (Genesis 25:21, Genesis 26:12-1) surely caused her faith to increase. Since we know she was a praying woman (Genesis 25:22, 23), I can assume that during these long years away from his family, Rebekah prayed for the safety of her beloved son. While we don't hear of Rebekah again after she sent Jacob away, we do know that her prayer for her son's safety was answered as he reunited in peace with his brother Esau (Genesis 33:4).

I want to remind you that you are not alone in your prayers for children. Your ancestors who might have been slaves, servants, crop sharers, indentured servants, or even nobility, etc., may have all at one point prayed for the blessing upon their future descendants. You may not have ever met them, but they have prayers that have been sent up to heaven on your behalf that God is waiting to answer. Whether that answer comes in the form of a biological child, adopted child, fostered child, niece, nephew, cousin, or mentee, God will answer not only your prayers but theirs. Think about it like this: by the time Abraham died, Isaac (the child through which nations would be built) and Rebekah only had two teenage sons. Abraham wasn't able to see the promise of nations in his lifetime, but because his assurance in God fulfilling His promises, he knew his prayers would be answered.

Keep praying, keep hoping, and walk in the assurance that God will answer the prayers of not only you, but your mother as well.

Things to Ponder...

1. Are there any prayers that you remember your parents praying over you? Have you witnessed them being fulfilled?

2. Have you reached out to talk to your parents and/or

in-laws about the challenges you and your spouse are facing in conception?

3. Have you thought about the other ways that God could be answering your call to parenthood? Have you prayed to see if God is calling you to adopt or foster?

Scriptures for Inspiration
Deuteronomy 29:13; Acts 26:6

DAY 17
Hidden Idols

Devotional Reading:
Genesis 31:18-35

Key Verse:
"And Laban went to shear his sheep: and Rachel had stolen the images that were her father's." – Genesis 31:19

Key Word Definitions:

Repent — feel or express sincere regret or remorse about one's wrongdoing or sin **and turn away**

Idol — an image or representation of a god used as an object of worship

After a few years of unsuccessful attempts at getting pregnant, my fertility challenges began to be noted by family members. While I have been extremely blessed to be a part of a large, extended, loving family, I have learned that not all good intentions have good outcomes. My family has prayed for and with my husband and me for fruitfulness, shared stories and testimonies of their own issues with conception and been an awesome support system. However, all support, while well-meaning, wasn't for me.

A well-meaning elder loaned me a fertility statue to keep close to my bed. She noted that she had heard testimonies from several people who were struggling to conceive, and once they had the fertility statue in their inner space they conceived. I felt a little uncomfortable taking the gift from the elder, but my desire to have a child was so strong that I let my desires overrule my uneasiness. I took possession of the statue and brought it home and knew immediately I had made an error in judgment. Not only had my uneasiness not dissipated, but I was ashamed to tell my husband because I knew his reaction would be, "Get it out of our home!"

I struggled with this for quite a long time. Fairly soon I realized that God had been speaking to me about this statue for a long time, I simply wasn't willing to listen. All of the uneasiness and shame I was experiencing was really the Holy Spirit's nudging and telling me to return the gift. Who knows if I was blocking my blessing from God because of the idol I had in my presence. Once I came to this realization, I didn't even have to figure a way to return it; the elder asked for it back. Most importantly, I repented for bringing this idol into my household.

Today's verse shares how Rachel, Jacob's beloved wife, took some images (idols) that belonged to her father when the family left Laban. These Scriptures provide words of warning that we should heed while on this journey.

1. **Even the strongest Christian can fall into old bad habits.** We know from Genesis 30:22 that Rachel called out to God because He heard her. While there hadn't been mention of idols in Laban's household before this verse, the Bible introduces this hidden part of Rachel's upbringing when she is now preparing to leave the comfort of her old life. I like to think that Rachel wasn't actively worshipping these idols;

however, when confronted with change, she fell back to her old habits. When confronted with change (i.e., an uncomfortable medical diagnosis, diminishing finances, etc.), don't fall back into habits from which you have been delivered. Keep your focus on God and your ears open to hear from Him.

2. **If you have to hide it, it's probably not right.** God has given us the gift of the Holy Spirit to help us to know right from wrong. Many things might seem innocent, such as yoga, acupuncture, and fertility statues, but they are actually avenues to let in other entities that can potentially fracture your relationship with God. The Holy Spirit serves as our gut check. If you are feeling uneasiness about a fertility avenue, stop and pray for guidance from the Holy Spirit, and FOLLOW HIS LEAD.

3. **Your sinful actions can cause an avalanche of crazy reactions.** By Rachel's stealing her father's idols, Laban came after her and Jacob. He accused Jacob of stealing and almost went to battle with him over her actions. If she had been caught, especially after Jacob had finished giving a long spiel about his honor and service to Laban, her actions would have ruined his testimony. When you allow yourself to get caught up in idol worship (because believing in anything other than God as the cause of your fertility success is worship), you could actually be damaging the testimony of your spouse or even yourself.

I ask that you learn from my experience. Before proceeding with any decision, activity, buying any product, bringing anything into your home, PRAY. Lean on God and God alone to direct you to the best path for your situation.

Things to Ponder...

1. Is there something that you are doing in pursuit of a child about which you feel ashamed?

2. What do you think the Holy Spirit is telling you about this item/issue?

3. What are some bad habits from which you have been delivered?

4. Have you repented for bringing bad spirits into your life?

Scriptures for Inspiration

Luke 1:25; John 16:8; Proverbs 24:24, 25; James 1:5; Proverbs 2:6; James 3:17

DAY 18
Building Muscles

Devotional Reading:
Genesis 32

Key Verses:
"And Jacob was left alone; and there wrestled a man with him until the breaking of the day. And when he saw that he prevailed not against him, he touched the hollow of his thigh; and the hollow of Jacob's thigh was out of joint, as he wrestled with him. And he said, Let me go, for the day breaketh. And he said, I will not let thee go, except thou bless me."
– Genesis 32:24-26

Key Word Definitions:

Wrestled — to take part in a fight, either as sport or in earnest, that involves grappling with one's opponent and trying to throw or force them to the ground; struggle with a difficult problem

Did you know that muscles are grown through damage repair?

As you work out doing intensive anaerobic exercises like weightlifting, your body responds by damaging the muscle fibers thus triggering the repair process. White blood cells rush to injured muscles and reduce inflammation, cytokine proteins are released that starts the production of satellite cells, and the satellite cells bind with existing muscle fibers and facilitate not only repair but growth. What's interesting to note is that all of this repair and growth work doesn't happen when you're actually working out; it happens during a period of rest.

In today's reading Jacob is getting ready to reunite with Esau after a twenty-year separation. The last time they had seen each other, Jacob had robbed Esau of his birthright as well as his father's specific blessing. Esau was incredibly upset and planned to kill Jacob as soon as their father died. Their mother Rebekah sent Jacob away, and he had been living outside the family ever since. During his journey home, anxiety regarding the impending meeting was starting to get to him. Even though Jacob had seen God move countless times on his behalf, when confronted with the news that Esau was traveling with 400 men to intercept him, he started to become fearful.

Jacob sends away his family and goes to a place where he can be alone. I like to think during this time of nervousness that he desires to be alone so that he can commune with God and get advice about how best to proceed. It's in this time of quietness he begins to wrestle with a man. A couple of thoughts came to my mind when reading the key verses.

1. **Jacob wrestled for a while.** It may seem like our challenge with successful conception may be lasting a while. For some of us, it's only been a few months while others have been trying to get pregnant for years. We can still have hope that dawn is coming. Have you ever wrestled with someone? No matter how strong and how good of shape you may be in, eventually your body will get physically tired. According to the Guinness World Records, the longest professional

wrestling match lasted twelve hours and consisted of six participants rotating in and out.[1] Jacob was alone and wrestled throughout the night. I'm sure he was tired and exhausted, yet he wasn't defeated because he refused to give up until he received what he was seeking.

2. **The angel prevailed not against him.** The man with whom Jacob was wrestling was an angel of the Lord. We know that Jacob was seeking guidance from God on how to approach and reestablish a relationship with his brother. Jacob refused to quit until he received his blessing from God (v. 29). God wants to use this period of wrestling to build up your muscles of faith. The more you engage and push your faith muscles while waiting to conceive, the closer you can draw to God and to receiving the blessing from Him that you seek.

3. **Jacob changed after his encounter with God**. During the wrestling process, the angel touched the hollow of Jacob's thigh, causing it to be permanently out of joint (vv. 31, 32). While you are going through this waiting process, God is working on changing the inner you. You are not only building your muscle of faith, but also the other parts of the fruit of the Spirit:

    a. **Love.** Your love for God is growing and can be seen in how you interact with your spouse, your other children, your extended support system, or others who are going through the same issues.

    b. **Joy.** Your soul will be filled with delight to help you handle any not-so-awesome news.

    c. **Peace.** Your anxiety and stress levels are decreasing because you are finding true rest in God.

    d. **Longsuffering**. Your mental and emotional strength to deal with difficult situations and decisions will increase.

- e. **Gentleness**. Your morals and values will change to align more with God's will as you spend more time in study and prayer.

- f. **Goodness**. You will be able to inspire others to want to know God with the spiritual wellness that you are displaying.

- g. **Meekness**. You will be able to humbly let others know that it's only because of God that you are able to persevere through this challenging time.

- h. **Temperance**. You will be able to exercise better self-control to help you make better decisions regarding your physical health to put you in the best position to receive this fertility blessing from God.

Once we've completed our time of wrestling with fertility, then it's time for us to rest in God's blessing (Matthew 11:28). Keep wrestling; even though you can't see it, your muscles are growing.

Things to Ponder...

1. For what specifically do you feel you need to wrestle with God?

2. Have you ever quit in the middle of a wrestling match with God? Why? What do you think you can do differently now to get a different outcome?

3. Do you feel yourself growing in your relationship with God during this time?

Scriptures for Inspiration
Psalm 30:5; Hosea 12:4

1. "Longest Professional Wrestling Match," Guinness World Records, accessed August 31, 2020, https://www.guinnessworldrecords.com/world-records/longest-match-professional-wrestling?.

DAY 19
Communication Is Key

Devotional Reading:
Genesis 34

Key Verse:
"And Jacob heard that he had defiled Dinah his daughter: now his sons were with his cattle in the field: and Jacob held his peace until they were come." – Genesis 34:5

Key Word Definitions:

Communication — the imparting or exchanging of information or news

Good communication is vital to enjoying a successful relationship. During this time of heightened emotional, physical, spiritual, and financial stress, making sure you and your spouse are communicating effectively is so important to keeping not only each of you well balanced but also encouraged. According to a study published in *Acta Obstetricia et Gynecologica Scandinavica*, women who do not have a child after fertility treatments were three times more likely to divorce than those who do. That's a super-intense fact, and I know that you are not aiming to become another number in those statistics.

Today's reading shares the tragedy that befalls Jacob's daughter Dinah. This young girl is kidnapped and violated by a prince of the land. When Jacob learns of this assault, he opts to withhold the information from his sons for a time. We aren't told the why of Jacob's actions, but we soon see the result in this fateful decision. His sons learn of her defilement through hearsay (v. 7), and in their anger, decide to mete out an extremely harsh punishment (vv. 13, 25-29). Perhaps if Jacob had told his sons sooner, they might not have reacted in a way that put their family in danger (v. 30) and displeased God (Genesis 35:1-4).

Talk with your husband regarding each other's thoughts and emotions during this time. Be honest about where your head is at so that issues aren't misinterpreted or frustrations aren't vented on the wrong person. Pray with each other and for each other. Take time out each day to go through the Bible together not only to find words of encouragement regarding your specific situation but also to remind yourself that God desires for you to have a beautiful, loving marriage "Let him kiss me with the kisses of his mouth: for thy love is better than wine," (Song of Solomon 1:2). God wants us to have a passionate marriage so, as hard as it may be, don't allow stress regarding conception to take the joy out of conceiving.

First Things First, a non-profit organization that provides affordable relationship resources to all, notes these few tips for improving the quality of your relationship.

- Be intentional about spending time talking together.
- Use more "I" statements and fewer "You" statements.
- Be specific.
- Avoid mindreading.
- Express negative feelings constructively.

- Listen without being defensive.
- Freely express positive feelings.

My husband and I could have used these tips when discussing the possibility of adoption. Instead of listening to his reasons for his initial decision of no, I let my own desire to become a mother close my ears to what he had to say. I started to not-so-subtly send him links to adorable kids looking to be adopted, told him of any children that I heard about who were in need of a home, and tried to set up lunch dates with other couples who had positive experiences to get him to change his mind. I would be present during our conversations about adoption, but once the word "no" would slip out of his mouth, I honestly would check out. It wasn't until I felt the nudge of the Holy Spirit telling me to pray about it that I realized my husband wasn't saying no, but was simply asking me to have patience to allow the Lord to guide our decision.

Remember that you aren't alone through this process. God has given you a loving spouse who wants to experience this joy with you as much as you do. Trust God to lead you through this journey together.

Things to Ponder...

1. What are some things that you think you need to improve upon to promote better communication with your spouse?
2. How can you let your spouse know what areas you want to work on together?
3. Are you caught up in the "mindreading" scenario? Do you think there are some matters that you need to clarify to make sure you fully understand each other's thoughts on a particular topic?

Scriptures for Inspiration
Psalm 115:6; Matthew 7:7; Acts 2:1; Ecclesiastes 4:9

DAY 20

By and By

Devotional Reading:
Genesis 36

Key Verse:
"Now these are the generations of Esau, who is Edom."
– Genesis 36:1

Key Word Definitions:
Unexplained — not described or made clear; unknown

Did you know that approximately twenty to thirty percent of couples who are having conception challenges have unexplained infertility? This statistic means that roughly a quarter (I'm averaging for simplicity) of the people who have difficulty getting pregnant will never have a definitive answer as to why. Have you received answers from medical professionals as to why you haven't been able to conceive?

While I have undergone the surgical procedure to remove the endometrial tissue that was taking over my body, I still have not been able to get pregnant. While roughly forty percent of women who have had the corrective surgery have subsequently gotten pregnant, I have not yet been blessed in that area. Studies have shown that the possibility of endometriosis resurfacing after surgery increases to almost fifty percent after five years. At the time of this writing, I am currently four years post-surgery, and without additional surgery, I am not sure if I'm in that elite group of women who have experienced resurgence since before my surgery, my symptoms were never quite noticeably severe.

All of this not knowing reminds me of today's reading. I know you're probably thinking, *Hey, Kel, how in the world are you going to tie Esau's lineage to a devotional about what to do while you're waiting to get pregnant?* When I read this chapter, I initially started creating a family tree for Esau. We know that every word in the Bible has a purpose (2 Timothy 3:16), but we also know that sometimes we don't immediately grasp the meaning. When I got to about verse fourteen and thought I was getting lost climbing up and down the tree, I stopped and asked God to give me insight as to why this particular lineage was important. Do you know what He answered?

"Just trust Me."

At this same time, a certain hymn started playing in my mind.

> *"We are often tossed and driv'n*
> *On the restless sea of time.*
> *Somber skies and howling tempests*
> *oft succeed a bright sunshine.*
> *In that land of perfect day,*
> *When the mists have rolled away,*
> *We will understand it better by and by."*

This hymn, "We'll Understand It Better By and By," by Charles Albert Tindley speaks to me on so many levels when I think about Genesis 36 and my own journey to motherhood. I definitely have times when I feel tossed and driven on this road to conception. When I hear negative reports from my doctors or "Aunt Flo" shows up (especially after being a week late), all I can see and hear are somber skies and howling tempests. What I love about this song is that it doesn't end with the restless sea or the somber skies but proceeds to let us know that a day will come when the mists (water droplets that limit visibility) will be rolled away. One day you and I will receive clarity about why we had to experience this journey, why we didn't get pregnant in our timing, why the process to become a mother was so hard, and what attribute God was trying to develop in us through this trial. One day I'll get the full understanding of why Esau's lineage was so important. It might not happen today, tomorrow, or a few years from now, but God always promises to provide understanding by and by.

Considerable anxiety can occur because we don't know the why or when of God's plan. I know it's hard, but I think in order to release the apprehension that we are feeling through this process, we need to change our pleas to God from "'Why, Lord, am I not pregnant yet?" to "Lord, please release the burden of why from my life and fill me with the contentment that only You can provide in ceding that only You know what's best."

Things to Ponder...

1. Are there some things for which you've been asking God to provide an explanation? How does it feel that He hasn't seemed to answer in the time frame you were looking for?

2. If we know God has a specific plan laid out for our lives (Jeremiah 29:11), why do you find it so hard to be patient in this plan? Are you struggling with the unknown?

Scriptures for Inspiration
Romans 8:28; Matthew 13:10-11; Proverbs 30:5; James 1:12; Job 12:22; Jeremiah 33:3

DAY 21
Jailbreak

Devotional Reading:
Genesis 39

Key Verses:
"And Joseph's master took him, and put him into the prison, a place where the king's prisoners were bound: and he was there in the prison. But the LORD was with Joseph, and shewed him mercy, and gave him favour in the sight of the keeper of the prison." – Genesis 39:20-21

Key Word Definitions:

Prison – a state of confinement or captivity
Captivity – held under control of another but having the appearance of independence
Bound – a limitation or restriction on feeling or action
Omnipresent – present everywhere at the same time

What image comes to mind when you think of the word prison? I think of grey, solid block walls, narrow, uncomfortable cots with thin, rough sheets, and a single toilet with no privacy and no toilet seat cover. In other words, I imagine a dark, cold, shame-filled place.

Sometimes our fertility struggles can make us feel like we're bound in a prison. The funny thing is, most of the times we are the ones who have bound ourselves. We limit our intimate activities to only "optimum" times, we restrict what types of clothing we may want to wear (boxers only so they can breathe), and we confine ourselves to following every piece of advice, whether or not medically proven, to the strict letter of the law all in our attempts to conceive a child. The restrictions can be downright depressing and exhausting!

In today's reading it's noted that Joseph has been sold into servitude. Potiphar, his master, saw how everything Joseph worked on was blessed, and soon he promoted him to be in charge of his entire household. The problem was Potiphar's wife also noticed how awesome Joseph was. She tried to seduce him and when he rebuked her advances, she lied about him to her husband, and Joseph was thrown into prison.

We can learn a few lessons from Joseph's prison experience that can be helpful in navigating our current condition.

1. **Joseph's situation was not his fault.** Your current situation is not your fault. No matter what people may say, especially family members whose well-meaning advice is often riddled with little barbs, fertility challenges are not a curse or a punishment for some previous sin that you may have committed. We must keep in mind that we serve a God who wants us to have life (in and out of the womb) and have it more abundantly (John 10:10). He wants us to be blessed so much that He sacrificed His Son for this to happen.

2. **Joseph's reaction to being in prison was purposeful.** Imagine if you were accused of a crime that you didn't commit and thrown into jail without any trial or opportunity to plead your case. I feel relatively sure

you'd be angry and bitter and sitting in some corner somewhere pouting, but Joseph chose instead to continue to do the work he was given. He continued to let God use him by interpreting the dreams of some of the king's closest workers (Genesis 40:8-19). And just as He did when Joseph found himself sold to Potiphar, God allowed him to flourish where he was.

What is your reaction to being in this situation of fertility uncertainty? Do you still wake up each morning with a grateful heart that is yearning after God's will instead of your will or have you let your invisible prison turn you away from God? Speak the words of Colossians 4:2 and 1 Thessalonians 5:16-18 each morning and night. Meditate on them continuously until the Holy Spirit makes thankfulness a reality in your life. Jesus has a plan for each and every one of us, and He wants us to keep the faith and not grow weary, because in due season... (See Galatians 6:9.)

3. **God doesn't want us in permanent bondage.** God sent His Son Jesus to live, die, and rise again so that we could be free from any and all bondage. I love how God reiterates twice that He was with Joseph (vv. 21, 23). Why do you think we are reminded again that God was with him? I believe the reminder is to point out that not only is God with us wherever we are, but that He is the One who allows us to flourish in no matter what situation we face! God can grant favor on us at any time and any place whether it's in the doctor's office, in the bedroom when you're up in the middle of the night wondering when your time will come, or as you're driving to pick up your new adopted son. He is omnipresent (Isaiah 57:15)!

Be heartened. In the midst of your "prison," God is there.

Things to Ponder...

1. Do you feel like your conception issues are a result of some previous sin you or your ancestor has committed? If so, why?

2. What is one thing that you believe God is telling you to do during this time of waiting? Seek God for confirmation on how you are to move in this place.

3. If God doesn't want us in bondage, why are we still creating fertility prisons for ourselves?

Scriptures for Inspiration
Isaiah 61:1; Jeremiah 30:10; 2 Corinthians 3:17

WEEK 4

Luteal Phase: Who's Your Bible Mentor?

After the follicle releases its egg, it changes into the corpus luteum. This structure releases hormones, mainly progesterone and some estrogen. The rise in hormones keeps your uterine lining thick and ready for a fertilized egg to implant. If you do get pregnant, your body will produce human chorionic gonadotropin (hCG). Pregnancy tests detect this hormone, which helps maintain the corpus luteum and keeps the uterine lining thick. If you don't get pregnant, the corpus luteum will shrink away and be reabsorbed, leading to decreased levels of estrogen and progesterone, which causes the onset of your period. The uterine lining will shed during your period.[1]

Mentor = an experienced and trusted adviser

As we enter this last phase of our journey, the waiting period has now begun. For me, this can be the hardest time. I go about my normal daily affairs but keep wondering if this will be the month of success. I tell myself not to get my hopes up because it's too soon to tell and even begin bargaining with God (that if I am not pregnant yet to work another divine miracle so that somehow the egg will meet the sperm.)

Whether you're in school, at work, a part of a non-profit organization or church ministry, one way to be successful is by having a mentor. A mentor not only helps guide you through difficult decisions based upon their own experiences, but can also help instruct and encourage you because the person has been where you are. While going through this journey of conception, I searched through the Bible to find whose experience was most similar to mine. I wanted to draw encouragement and wisdom from the person as I read her story and saw how she handled her "meantime." I found that Elisabeth's story most resonated with me for three reasons:

1. She **experienced** the same issue with conception as me.

2. She could be **trusted** due to her character as described by Luke.

3. I could look to her as an **adviser** to know how to walk during this journey.

As the pastor would announce, "Take out your Bible and turn to the book of Luke..." but before getting into the story of Elisabeth, I want to preface my thoughts by saying that this book of the Bible was written by Luke, a physician (Colossians 4:14). I think Luke's vocation is important to note because, for the first time, the story of a couple challenged with fertility issues is told from the eyes of a doctor. While most babies at that time were delivered by midwives, physicians were still somewhat knowledgeable about the normal functions of the human body. To me, Luke's description of barrenness takes on a more official feeling—especially since I've had doctors tell me the number of remaining eggs will likely prohibit my being able to conceive.

I learned a few key takeaways from Elisabeth's story that I have begun to incorporate in my life to give me hope and increase my faith.

Even though she and her husband, Zacharias, lived a righteous life before God, Elisabeth was still barren. Because we know that Jesus is the only living person who ever lived a completely righteous life, what Luke 1:6 is telling us is that this couple purposely and daily attempted to do God's will outwardly, and most importantly, inwardly in their hearts. Yet Elisabeth was still barren (v. 7).

I think it's important to note that the Word specifically calls out that their childlessness was due to Elisabeth. The conception stories covered throughout this study of Genesis have never particularly called out any men as being the cause of fertility challenges. When researching how barrenness was viewed back in Biblical times, I came across *Matthew Henry's Commentary* on Luke 1, which stated the following:

> Fruitfulness was looked upon to be so great a blessing amoung the Jews, because of the promise of the increase of

their nation, and the rising of the Messiah amoung them, that it was a great reproach to be barren; and those who were so, though ever so blameless, were concluded to be guilty of some great sin unknown, for which they were punished.²

Not only was it known that the cause of their childlessness was due to Elisabeth's physical problems, but she also knew that people were probably ridiculing her and/or judging her behind her back during this especially sensitive time in her life. And the couple had braved the judgments a long time since we know from Luke 1:7 that she was now well stricken in years.

In both of these circumstances, I can feel Elisabeth's pain. For me in my journey, medical tests conducted on my husband and myself pointed to my body being the most likely cause of our conception challenges. In addition, for every year that has gone by without successful conception, I have felt a deeper sense of shame since I haven't been able to carry on the Ferguson family name. While in today's time it's not as great of a stigma to see childless women, we are still constantly asked why we don't have any and are sometimes thought of as being too selfish to desire to carry on as nature intended.

I remember when my husband and I were dating, and I was conversing with his mom about the upcoming birth of my now-nephew. She was so excited that her son and daughter-in-law were having another boy. Up until that point, I had always wanted to have little girls and couldn't understand her exuberance over a boy in particular. She told me to know that the Ferguson family name was going to continue on excited her. My mother-in-law passed away a little more than a year before we were married. Even though I know in my heart that she would be happy for our strong, loving marriage of ten years, I can't also help but think she would be disappointed that I haven't been able to add to her grandchildren count. *Would she wonder if my husband should have married someone else?*

They didn't let their current circumstance stop them from doing the work of God. Both Zacharias and Elisabeth were known for "walking" in all the commandments of the Lord (v. 6). *Walking* indicates that they were moving, busy, doing. They weren't standing around moping about their situation or wallowing in frustration that God would put this burden of childlessness on them. They kept active in doing God's will.

Through my journey I've found myself more active in studying God's Word and increasing my prayer life. While I'm waiting on God's answer, I've started to develop more of the attributes that God is calling us to have such as patience, long-suffering, hope and faith. My heart has been filled with more joy over baby announcements now than before when a bit of envy and anger would pop up since it wasn't my turn. I have learned that God really does speak to me in the quiet times and that gives me strength to go out and execute for Him.

Because of their intimate relationship with God, Zacharias rightly discerned an angel of God was speaking about the specifics of their upcoming blessing. Can you imagine what that must have been like for him? An old man who had probably given up on the idea of having a child is now being told that God is going to answer his prayers. Not only is his blessing coming, but the angel described in specific detail what John would be like. Now, even though Zacharias was a praying, believing man of God, it's understandable that he questioned the angel for proof (v. 18). Why would a priest who knew of the miracles of Isaac, Jacob, and Joseph's births react this way? I believed he reacted for the same reason I would react if someone came and told me I was going to be pregnant with twins. Fearful! I think Zacharias asked for confirmation not out of doubting God's ability to make it happen, but out of fear that he and Elisabeth were actually chosen for this miracle. Have you ever been a bit nervous or scared when something too good to be true is presented to you? If so, I believe you can understand how Zacharias felt.

As soon as Zacharias got home, he got to work. Elisabeth conceived immediately following the angel's pronouncement.

When God decides to move, it will happen quickly and without delay (Habakkuk 2:3). But Elisabeth conceived only because Zacharias made a move. There was only one divine conception in history; therefore, in order for God's Word to manifest, Elisabeth and Zacharias had to actually put in the work. Are you praying for a child but not actively engaging in intimate relations with your husband? We don't know whether or not Elisabeth conceived after one time, but hey, you can't ever get enough practice!

Elisabeth praised God upon conception. The Word tells us that for five months Elisabeth hid herself away (v. 25). While modern-day customs tell women to keep silent for the first trimester for fear of miscarriage, I don't think that this was the reason Elisabeth stayed secluded. This was a time of rejoicing and celebration for her of God's promise fulfilled. I think that she isolated herself in order to remove negative influence from her space (i.e., the people always looking down upon her). During this sacred time in her life, she wanted to spend as much time as possible staying connected to God so that she would have the strength to make it through this pregnancy with her mind, body, and spirit intact. Remember that Elisabeth wasn't a young girl, and her body would need some extra attention to make sure she had a healthy delivery.

Getting your physical health in order during the meantime so that you have the best housing available for your hopeful "tenant" is important. Not only that, don't make your praise a one-day event. You should be continuously praising God throughout this process for who He is, what He has done, and what He will do.

Sometimes your delay is for a bigger purpose. God's timing is perfect (Ecclesiastes 3:1). If John had not been conceived at that specific time, Elisabeth would not have been pregnant to bring confirmation of the angel Gabriel's words to Mary (Luke 1:36). Elisabeth's pregnancy brought comfort to Mary in her own miracle time. If Elisabeth, who was well past child-bearing years, could be pregnant after receiving a word from the Lord, then God would fulfill His Word to a young Mary about the babe she was carrying. If I hadn't experienced this delay in conception/adoption/mentoring, etc., I would not have written this book, which is hopefully helping you through your own journey and drawing you closer to God.

As we enter into the final phase of our menstrual cycle, I want to encourage you to find a mentor in the Bible who speaks to your specific circumstance. Do you feel drawn to the experiences of Sarah (Genesis 11:30), Rebekah (Genesis 25:21), Rachel (Genesis 29:31), Samson's mother (Judges 13:2) or Hannah (1 Samuel 1:5)? Take joy in knowing that God can make the barren woman a joyful mother to children (Psalm 113:9). God is speaking to you through His Word. Are you listening?

1. Stephanie Watson, "Stages of the Menstrual Cycle," healthline, updated August 7, 2018, https://www.healthline. com/health/womens-health/stages-of-menstrual-cycle#luteal.

2. Matthew Henry, Matthew Henry Study Bible-King James Version, (Nashville: Thomas Nelson, Inc., 1991566.

DAY 22

The Importance of Warming Up

Devotional Reading:
Genesis 39:2-6, 21-23; Genesis 41:36-44

Key Verse:
"Then Pharaoh sent and called Joseph, and they brought him hastily out of the dungeon: and he shaved himself, and changed his raiment, and came in unto Pharaoh."
– Genesis 41:14

Key Word Definition:
Training — the action of teaching a person or animal a particular skill or type of behavior

I have already mentioned spending months training for a 10K. For some people, running 6.2 miles is rather easy. They either already participate in other athletic sports and/or are naturally more physically fit than others. Running for me was not something that I could simply put on some tennis shoes and just start. Readying myself for this run required a slow build-up of my stamina and confidence so that I would be able to handle the challenge. The training caused me to be vulnerable in front of friends and strangers, finding out that some people are willing to help push and encourage you to keep pressing on. The training made me reach deep inside, especially when my lungs started to burn and sweat was dripping in my eyes, to find the source of strength from God to keep putting one foot in front of the next. Running my race wasn't pretty or record breaking, but the training I endured helped me cross the finish line all those months later.

I know that the reason why you are reading this devotional is because somewhere deep inside, you want to have a child or children. While you are believing in God for your miracle, are you also taking the time to prepare for the blessing to come? Are you activating your faith by putting in work to help you improve yourself in the following ways?

- Learning how to change a diaper

- Gaining patience because kids will test you in ways you can't even imagine

- Learning how to go with the flow because a baby doesn't cry on a schedule

- Learning how to make basic meals because kids need proper nutrition

- Learning how to set aside specific time for your spouse; no if, ands, or buts because keeping your marriage strong goes a long way to co-parenting in a healthy way

In the devotional reading today, examples of how God prepared Joseph for his role as Pharaoh's governor are addressed. As a servant, he learned how to manage the affairs of Potiphar's house with so much success that his master didn't worry about anything except what food he would be eating—not if there was food, but how much of it to consume. As a prisoner, Joseph continued to develop his management skills while being in charge of his fellow prisoners. He stretched his God-faith muscles by not only reaching out to show empathy for the baker and the butler, but by also being willing to interpret their dreams—even when the news wasn't completely rosy. All this work was preparing him for not only interpreting Pharaoh's dream correctly, but also having the knowledge to expertly articulate what Pharaoh should do to prevent the famine from affecting his nation.

We can take heed of Joseph's example and use this time of waiting to develop some of the skills that motherhood requires. I had the wonderful opportunity to babysit my nieces when they were really small. I hadn't had a lot of experience with babies at this point and was just trying to do my best and follow the instructions laid out by my sister. Unfortunately, I didn't know that when making formula you aren't supposed to use cow's milk! Thankfully, my niece suffered no serious aftereffects during this "training" process for me. A few years later as I started to get closer to my IVF treatment dates, I realized that I was going to need to definitely brush up on my "mommy" skills. I joined my church's nursery ministry and have been so blessed because of that decision. Not only do I know how to quickly and efficiently change a stinky diaper and how to use a bottle warmer, but I got to spend more time around little people just basking in all their amazing uniqueness.

What are some steps you can take to train for this never-ending job of motherhood? I want to encourage you to think about nontraditional ways to increase your mommy skills. Have you thought about volunteering as a mentor? What about joining the children's ministry at your church? Do you know of any friends and/or family members who have little ones and could use a night out? We can't prepare for everything, but God is asking us to show our faith in Him by putting our words into actions (James 2:14).

Things to Ponder...

1. What experiences with children have you had?
2. Do you think that God can use your previous experiences to make you a better mother?
3. To what will you commit in order to help you broaden your "mommy" skills?

Scriptures for Inspiration
James 2:14-26

DAY 23

Fruitful in the Land of Affliction

Devotional Reading:
Genesis 39:2-6, 21-23; Genesis 41:36-44

Key Verses:
"And the name of the second called he Ephraim: For God hath caused me to be fruitful in the land of my affliction."
– Genesis 41:52

"And he said, Behold, I have heard that there is corn in Egypt: get you down thither, and buy for us from thence; that we may live, and not die." – Genesis 42:2

Key Word Definitions:
Fruitful — producing much fruit; fertile; producing good or helpful results; productive
Affliction — something that causes pain or suffering

It's time to talk about money. I know finances can be an

uncomfortable subject to address, but it's real, it's necessary and at some point, has to be considered. While discussing your family growth options, make sure to take time out with your spouse to review all costs associated with each option. Whether you conceive naturally, through fertility assistance, choose to adopt or foster, costs can be associated with each option.

During this time of waiting, God is giving you the opportunity to prepare for the blessings to come. He is asking us to be fruitful in this time of affliction. In our reading for today, we see the culmination of Joseph's time of affliction. He was mistreated by his brothers, sold into servitude, thrown into a prison and now has been promoted from prisoner to governor. This prison-to-the-palace process didn't take place overnight. Joseph's life of normalcy stopped when he was only seventeen (Genesis 37:2). Not until he was thirty (Genesis 41:4) was he presented with the divine opportunity to have his life transformed yet again. He experienced thirteen years of wondering how God was going to make a way. Have you been waiting thirteen months for a positive sign on the pregnancy test stick? Five years? Thirteen years? But the wonder of Joseph's story during this time is he still worked and gained the mindset of what was needed to be successful in whatever path God planned for him.

Famine did come to the land as Joseph had prophesized. The key takeaway is that while Jacob may not have been storing up corn and crops during the seven years of plenty, he still didn't mishandle his finances. During the good times, he was knowledgeable enough to learn to save in order to be able to have funds to be able to purchase corn from Egypt. How would a downturn in the economy affect your finances? Would your savings that were set aside for fertility treatments be consumed for necessities, thus delaying that option? How are you preparing your finances to account for the costs it takes to adopt? Are you seeking God for wisdom in regard to every aspect of your parenthood story?

The following are some quick facts about what it takes financially to become a parent[1,2,3]:

- IUI Treatment = $500 – $4,000
- IVF Treatment = $20,000
- Hospitalization for Natural Birth in US = $5,000 – $11,000
- Hospitalization for C-section Birth in US = $7,500 – $14,500
- First-Year Cost of Diapers/Wipes = $1,100
- International Adoption = $36,000 – $46,000
- Domestic Adoption = $34,000 – $40,000
- Foster Adoption = $3,000

Wow! Talk about a lot to digest! My husband and I went through a similar exercise when we started our IVF treatments. Due to my history with endometriosis, IUI wasn't an option the specialist could recommend for us. Thank goodness for excellent insurance! Because my husband's employer had great benefits, we were allowed up to a maximum of two tries for IVF before we would have to pay out of pocket. I had good insurance with the company that I worked for; however, fertility treatments were not included. (Be sure to always read the fine print.) I cannot even imagine how our conversation would have gone had we not had insurance to cover the costs, especially since both trials didn't result in a pregnancy for us.

If you are unsure of how to proceed, please take the time to pray. The Bible contains many great nuggets of wisdom regarding finances that you should check out for inspiration. Pray the Scriptures, i.e., recite God's Word back to Him and watch how He'll give you insight on how to move forward.

Things to Ponder...

1. Do you regularly talk about money with your spouse? Do you understand your household's finances?

2. Do you have a separate savings set up for conception expenses?

3. Have you reviewed your insurance coverage language to see what treatments are covered?

Scriptures for Inspiration

Philippians 4:19; Proverbs 22:7; Proverbs 3:9; Luke 14:28-30; Luke 16:11

---

1. Rickie Houston, "Average Cost of Having a Baby in 2019," October 18, 2019, https://smart asset.com/financial-advisor/cost-of-having-a-baby.

2. "Cost of IVF: Cost Components," Fertility IQ, assessed August 31, 2020, https://www.fertilityiq.com/ivf-in-vitro-fertilization/costs-of-ivf#cost-components.

3. Eva Dasher, "First-Year Baby Costs Calculator," Baby Center, LLC, Updated July 23, 2020, https://www.babycenter.com/baby-cost-calculator.

DAY 24

Healing Tears

Devotional Reading:
Genesis 42: 6-8, 24; 43:27-30; 45:1-5

Key Verses:
"Then Joseph could not refrain himself before all them that stood by him; and he cried, Cause every man to go out from me. And there stood no man with him, while Joseph made himself known unto his brethren. And he wept aloud: and the Egyptians and the house of Pharaoh heard."
– Genesis 45:1-2

Key Word Definitions:
Refrain — to contain, restrain
Wept — to call aloud; a voice or sound; bleating, crackling; cry out, yell

My father passed away unexpectedly when I was twenty-six years old. At the time, my younger sister was still in college, I was working fulltime but had not learned good money management, and my dad and stepmom had been divorced for six months. I was filled with a profound sense of grief and stressed beyond belief with all the responsibilities thrust upon my shoulders. I didn't feel like I could show how overwhelmed I felt; after all, my sister was depending on me. While we had extended family and friends surrounding us with support, at the end of the day, I felt like it was just the two of us staring at a pile of invoices for a funeral we didn't know how to plan with limited time and resources. In a span of five days I went from having a father who would smile through my humble cooking attempts to trying to figure out why there's separate costs to open and close a burial plot. I didn't see it coming, couldn't figure out how to healthily process my emotions, and as a result, ended up with a stomach ulcer.

We've all been in situations where grief has threatened to drown us. Maybe it was due to a failed fertility procedure, a bad report from a doctor, a pregnancy that didn't go to term, or an adoption process that didn't come to fruition. No matter the reason, I want to let you know that it's okay to feel any and everything, but don't let it break you.

In the reading today Joseph is overcome with emotions when he is reunited with his brothers after twenty years apart. Although Joseph has been in constant fellowship with God, when confronted with an unexpected encounter, he is overcome. We don't know if Joseph was crying out with gladness to be back with his family or releasing pent-up anger and bitterness from seeing the faces of those he loved who had sold him into slavery. No matter what the reason, we know that all of the constrained emotions he had buried within himself burst out like a geyser—at inopportune times. Isn't it funny how we often think that we've dealt with a situation/emotion/circumstance and have moved on only to get checked quickly when confronted with something that brings those old memories back to the surface?

A study done by the Harvard School of Public Health and the University of Rochester found that suppressing emotions may increase the risk of dying from heart disease and certain forms of cancer.[1] In other words, locking down your emotions in order to put on a happy face and not make others uncomfortable with your situation (i.e., Grandma's best friend who keeps asking when you're going to have kids), or trying to speed up the healing process is not only hurting your spiritual heart but your physical one also. While my stomach ulcer wasn't a disease of the heart, I can tell you that during my time of mourning, I could physically feel my heart hurting.

I want to encourage you to take a real good look within yourself and see if you have any locked-up residual emotions just waiting to be released. While tears truly do heal, I am asking you to seek God in prayer, be honest, and unburden your heart. Our God is loving, kind and ever so compassionate that He specializes in healing hearts. The prescription to our heart hurts is in the Word and our prayer time with God. It might not be immediate, but each day it will get better.

I'll always miss my dad, but now I can look back at the time we had together with happiness and gratefulness.

Things to Ponder...

1. Name something over which you have grieved. It doesn't necessarily have to be a loved one.

2. What ways have you tried to handle your grief? Were they short-term solutions or something that brought permanent peace?

3. What does it mean to you to hear the phrase "peace beyond understanding" (Philippians 4:7)?

4. Are you willing to surrender your grief to achieve God's peace?

Scriptures for Inspiration
Psalm 34:18; Psalm 147:3; Psalm 73:26; John 14:27; Psalm 55:22

1. Timi Gustafson, "Keeping Your Emotions Bottled Up Could Kill You," Huffington Post, March 31, 2014, https://www.huffingtonpost.ca/timi-gustafson/bottling-up-negative-emotions_b_ 5056433. html.

DAY 25
Feasting in the Famine

Devotional Reading:
Genesis 37:5-11; 45:4-28

Key Verse:
"And there I will nourish thee; for yet there are five years of famine; lest thou, and thy household, and all that thou hast, come to poverty." – Genesis 45:11

Key Word Definitions:
Nourish — provide with the food or other substances necessary for growth, health, and good condition

No matter how proactive, organized and detailed you are, there will be times when you will experience a season of famine. We talked earlier about what you are doing to prepare for your famine season (Days 22 and 23). Today's reading focuses on what seems to be God's reaction to your famine season that is really His proactive plan.

Have you ever read a book or watched a movie where at the

end of the grand reveal, you realize that the author/creator had been giving clues all along? One of my favorite movies of all time is the 1985 version of *Clue*. The movie, based on the board game, follows the antics of a group of strangers who meet for a formal dinner at a mysterious host's house only to be present when a murder (or multiple murders) are committed, and the group of strangers have to solve the crime(s). I laugh continuously throughout this movie at the crazy antics and personalities of all of the characters, but my favorite part is the end when the murderer is revealed. Why? Because one of the main suspects tells how seemingly insignificant clues of information have been given throughout the night to shine light on the eventual culprit.

God's Word is telling of a similar story today.

Clue 1. In Genesis 37, young Joseph dreamed dreams given to him by God. In these dreams, he is metaphorically shown that one day he will grow in stature (not so much in height but in power), and his family will bow down to him. This dream was so hard for his parents and brothers to hear because it was not customary for the son to rule over the father, and Joseph was the eleventh brother. Typically, the wealth and power would go to the eldest—not the youngest.

Clue 2. Joseph's brothers are not with their flocks in the location they were supposed to be. Jacob sends Joseph to look for his brothers in Shechem but when he catches up to them, they have moved to Dothan. I did a little research and noticed that Dothan is actually closer to the Great Sea than Shechem. While I couldn't find a definitive path that the Midianite travelers, who bought Joseph from his brothers, would typically take, I do know that they were desert dwellers and probably loved to experience a bit of the sea as often as their journeys would allow. If Joseph's brothers had stayed in Dothan, they most likely wouldn't have come across the Midianites, and perhaps Reuben would have had the opportunity to save him.

Clue 3. Joseph was sold into the household of Potiphar, Pharaoh's officer. During his wrongful imprisonment in this house, he had the chance to meet Pharaoh's chief butler (his executive assistant) and demonstrate how God could use him to interpret dreams. After all, he's been having them since he was at least seventeen years old. Later that same chief butler would bring him to the attention of Pharaoh, thus allowing God's intervention to put him in the position of Pharaoh's governor.

Mystery Solved. In Genesis 45, Joseph has revealed himself to his brothers and told them he now realizes that God's divine plan was for him to be in a position to help them through this time of famine.

During your famine season, what nourishment (i.e., spiritual guidance) is God providing for you based on the clues that He has already displayed? Are you being fed with encouragement from the stories of women in the Bible who have gone through similar circumstances? Are you filling your belly with faith and confidence in knowing that God will keep His Word? God will keep you during this journey to parenthood. Whether it's five years, seven years, or longer, He'll always be with you, making sure you have everything you need to thrive.

Things to Ponder...

1. Name one piece of "nourishment" God has given you to feast on during this famine?

2. What are some clues that God has given you, either from His Word or through the testimonies of others, to help you know that He is faithful and always there?

Scriptures for Inspiration
2 Corinthians 9:8; 2 Peter 1:3; Luke 12:24

DAY 26
Restoration of What Was Lost

Devotional Reading:
Genesis 46:1-5; 47:1-6, 27

Key Verse:
"I will go down with thee into Egypt; and I will also surely bring thee up again: and Joseph shall put his hand upon thine eyes." – Genesis 46:4

Key Word Definitions:
Restoration — the action of returning something to a former owner, place or condition

I have to be honest. Miscarriage is probably the most difficult topic for me to address because I have not personally experienced this situation. Perhaps for you, this day may be the hardest for you to get through because you have or are currently experiencing this loss. Addressing this subject can be difficult, but I think that healing comes in speaking your hurts out loud, especially to God. Just as God heard the cry of Ishmael when he was huddled beneath a bush in the desert, He hears and feels all of the pain, frustration, and anger that you are going through as you experience your miscarriage.

The Mayo Clinic defines *miscarriage* as the spontaneous loss of a pregnancy before the twentieth week.[1] I find so many things wrong with just reading that clinical definition.

- *Mis* is defined as a prefix meaning "ill, mistaken, wrong, incorrectly, negating." No child is ever a mistake. Psalm 127:3 tells us that children are one type of inheritance from God. Why would our God, who only gives good gifts (Matthew 7:11), ever give us something that is a mistake?

- *Carriage* is defined as "the transporting of items or merchandise from one place to another." To me this word minimizes the importance of the time in the womb for both mother and child. I can transport my purse in my car from one destination to another, but I will not give it the same care and attention as I would transporting my nieces or nephews. Carrying a child is about more than simply making sure that the infant stays in the belly. It's also about making sure the growing baby is getting the right nutrients by the choices you make regarding eating, making sure you remain calm and in a peaceful state so that that atmosphere transfers to the baby, etc.

Losing a child, no matter what the cause, is a loss that can be devastating if you let it swallow you whole. I cannot imagine the hurt of finally seeing a positive sign on the pregnancy test result only to have the very thing you've been hoping and praying for snatched away before you even get the chance to meet the infant.

In our reading today, we see that Jacob, while not experiencing a miscarriage, is still dealing with the loss of his beloved

Joseph more than twenty years later. He is so wrapped up in his grief that he almost costs the lives of his other children and people of his household by initially refusing to allow his sons to journey back to Egypt for the very food that will sustain them (Genesis 42:36-38). Is your grief crippling you from seeing the other opportunities that God is trying to show you?

When Jacob's sons return to share in the news that Joseph is still alive, at first, Jacob is in disbelief. While going through the motions to get ready to go to Egypt, he returns to where both his grandfather Abraham and his father Isaac made compacts with King Abimelech and praised the name of God. As a random side note, remember that King Abimelech's household had also suffered from barrenness. At this same place where once stood folks who all dealt with barrenness in one form or another, God was now about to speak to Jacob about the upcoming restoration of his son Joseph into his life!

Jacob will never get back the time that he lost being separated from Joseph. He'll never see him fall in love, witness his wedding, or be there to pat his back after the birth of his grandchildren. However, God blesses Jacob with the chance to live out the balance of his days in utter peace and joy. He is not only reunited with Joseph (Genesis 48:11), but he is brought to Egypt in style and treated as royalty.

You may not have been able to meet the little angel that God blessed you with for a short time, but that does not mean that you won't be blessed with more children or that your life won't be able to be full of joy once again. Our key verse reminds us not to be afraid of this next leg of the journey because God is with us.

Things to Ponder...

1. How are you dealing with the loss of your child?

2. Are you sharing your feelings with your spouse? With God?

3. What one Scripture can you memorize today to help bring you an expectation of hope that this too shall pass?

Scriptures for Inspiration
Matthew 5:4; Psalm 34:18; 2 Corinthians 1:3-4

1. "Miscarriage," Mayo Clinic, July 16, 2019, https://www.mayoclinic.org/diseases-conditions/ pregnancy-loss-miscarriage/symptoms-causes/syc-20354298.

DAY 27
Unexpected Blessings

Devotional Reading:
Genesis 48

Key Verse:
"And his father refused, and said, I know it, my son, I know it: he also shall become a people, and he also shall be great: but truly his younger brother shall be greater than he, and his seed shall become a multitude of nations." – Genesis 48:19

Key Word Definitions:
Unexpected — not regarded as likely to happen

When I was car shopping years ago, I knew in my heart the make and model of the vehicle I wanted. I had fallen in love with the 2012 Ford Escape and could even visualize myself behind the wheel. At the time of my search however, Ford had decided to change the body type of the Escape and had just introduced the 2013 model. My husband showed me pictures of the updated version, and I hated it! He couldn't even convince me to take a test drive at the dealership because it was so not my taste.

But God had other plans. The current car that I was driving at the time went kaput, and we were forced to have to make a quick decision on what to get in order to not interrupt our busy work lives too much. We went to the dealership that weekend with the intent to drive out in a 2012 model but ended up getting the last vehicle I expected—the 2013 Escape. I test drove the one single 2013 model that was in the lot because they were selling like hot cakes. Guess what? I fell in love! I did a complete 180° and we signed on the dotted line that afternoon. Want to know a secret? We even saved some money because the 2013 was slightly cheaper than the 2012 models at the time. Win, win!

This story popped in my mind when studying today's reading. How often have you found yourself in a similar situation of expecting one type of blessing but being surprised and excited about the course correction God had planned? Genesis 48 tells how Joseph brought his two sons to his father Jacob to bless before his passing. As per the customs of the time, the eldest son would always receive the first and best blessing. What happened instead is that Jacob intentionally placed the greater blessing upon the younger son's head. While Joseph was upset at this change in procedure, Jacob reassured him that one person's blessing doesn't negate another's. Indeed, both of his sons were blessed with greatness in numbers and power; only the younger would receive a greater amount.

Maybe you are looking at your current situation and asking God, "Why haven't You chosen to bless me in the way I expected? Why have others been favored with multiple children, and I haven't even had one?" Stay heartened because as the saying goes, God is still in the blessing business. While your prayers for having children may be answered in an unexpected way, have faith that God is going to answer in the way that He knows is best.

Things to Ponder...

1. Can you think of any unexpected blessings that you received in your life?

2. Are you thanking God for blessing you even if it's not the way that you desired to be blessed?

Scriptures for Inspiration

2 Corinthians 9:8; Jeremiah 17:7-8; 1 Kings 17:7-24

DAY 28

Temporary Space

Devotional Reading:
Genesis 47:27-31; 48:21; 50:25

Key Verse:
"And Israel said unto Joseph, Behold, I die: but God shall be with you, and bring you again unto the land of your fathers." – Genesis 48:21

Key Word Definitions:
Temporary — lasting only for a limited period of time; **not permanent**

Early in my career I was given the opportunity to move to Phoenix from Detroit for a temporary assignment. I was nervous and anxious not only because I would be working with a new team I had never met, but also because I would be living away from my family and anything remotely familiar for the first time in my life. The assignment was supposed to last anywhere from three to four weeks to help get another project started. I was just coming off one project without anything else lined up, so this opportunity seemed perfect for me to spread my trembling wings and fly.

Four weeks quickly turned into eight and when asked if I wanted to make the transfer permanent, I said yes. I had fallen in love with the Grand Canyon State, although ironically, I still haven't been to the Grand Canyon even until this day. What started out as completely uncomfortable and unfamiliar territory turned into a true appreciation for 100-plus degree days, sunshine so bright you just have to smile, majestic mountain views that put you in awe of God's goodness, and much, much more.

I ended up living in Phoenix for a little over two years. Although I flourished while planted there, ultimately it was only a temporary stop in my life's journey. God used my time in Phoenix to teach me to be comfortable in the quiet times, enjoy myself as company, and learn that I can accomplish new things if I put my mind to the task.

In our final reading, we discover how both Jacob and Joseph knew that their time in Egypt was only temporary. Although God had blessed them tremendously where they were, they knew that the place they truly wanted to be was in God's Promised Land. During your conception journey, while you may not be increasing your family size at this time, God is still blessing, enlarging, and positioning you for greater things to come. That promotion at work you just got could be His way of helping you to prepare for future daycare costs. That disappointing news the doctor just gave you is giving you the wisdom and tools to be able to step into the ministry leadership role you've been called to do. Don't believe that Egypt is the final destination when Canaan is right around the corner! I encourage you today to keep seeking God through prayer and the study of His Word so when your meantime is over you'll be ready to walk in the calling of motherhood, businesswoman, ministry leader, or whatever else God has specifically planned for you.

Be blessed in Jesus' holy name!

Things to Ponder...

1. What can you take away from your "meantime" experience?

2. During the course of these last twenty-eight days, what is one thing that has stood out to you to show you God's love for barren women?

3. What are some ways that you can minister to others who are going through a similar situation in order to help them draw closer to God?

Scriptures for Inspiration
Lamentations 3:24-25; Isaiah 30:18; James 5:7-8; 2 Peter 3:9

Afterword

I want to conclude this study by encouraging you to find your own personal battle song. For me the song that continues to inspire me on my journey is "Way Maker" by Sinach. If you can, I encourage you to listen to the song and start believing the words deep in your heart. God truly is a way maker, a miracle worker, a promise keeper, and a light in the darkness. His Word is true and will never *not* be fulfilled (Isaiah 55:11). God's desire is for us all to be fruitful and not barren (1 Samuel 2:5). I am believing in faith this word for myself and will continue to believe this for you as well. I cannot wait to hear the testimonies of how God has performed miracles in your lives. God bless!

Reference List

Week 1
Menstrual Phase: And Another One

Watson, Stephanie. 2019. "Stages of the Menstrual Cycle." *Healthline.*
https://www.healthline.com/health/womens-health/stages-of-menstrual-cycle#menstrual.

Day 3
Check the Receipts!

National Council for Adoption. 2014. "Choosing an Adoption Agency."
http://www.adoptioncouncil.org/ expectant-parents/find-an-agency.

Castaneda, Ruben. 2018. "How to Find a Good Fertility Clinic." *U.S. News and World Report.* https://health.usnews.com/health-care/patient-advice/articles/2018-04-30/how-to-find-a-good-fertility-clinic.

Howley, Elaine K. 2018. "How Can I Find the Best OB-GYN?" *U.S. News and World Report.*

https://health.usnews.com/health-care/patient-advice/articles/how-can-i-find-the-best-ob-gyn.

Day 4
A Dormant Branch

Blackstone, Victoria Lee. 2020. "Difference Between Dead & Dormant Branches," SF*Gate*. https://homeguides.sfgate.com/difference-between-dead-dormant-branches-85029.html#:~:text=Dormant%20branches%20are%20simply%20resting,are%20dead%20or%20simply%20dormant.

Day 7
Forgiveness = Healing

John Hopkins Medicine. 2020. "Forgiveness: Your Health Depends on It." https://www.hopkinsmedicine.org/health/wellness-and-prevention/forgiveness-your-health-depends-on-it.

Levine, Hallie. 2020. "How Stress Can Hurt Your Chances of Having a Baby," *Grow by Web* MD. https://www.webmd.com/baby/features/infertility-stress#1.

Week 2
Follicular Phase: Building Hope

Watson, Stephanie. 2019. "Stages of the Menstrual Cycle," *Healthline*.

https://www.healthline.com/health/womens-health/stages-of-menstrual-cycle#follicular.

Day 11
Having God's Ear

Orr, James, Editor. 1939. "Cleave." *The International Standard Bible Encyclopedia Online*. Grand Rapids: Wm. B. Eerdmans Publishing Co. https://www.internationalstandardbible.com/C/cleave.html.

Day 13
God's Strategic Power: Cracking Open the Jar

Martinelli, Katherine. 2012. "In a pickle: How to open a stuck jar," *SheKnows*.
https://www.sheknows.com/food-and-recipes/articles/963722/in-a-pickle-how-to-open-a-stuck-jar/.

Week 3
Ovulation Phase: Execution Time!

Watson 2019. https://www.healthline.com/health/womens-health/stages-of-menstrual-cycle#follicular.

Day 18
Building Muscles

Guinness World Records. 2020. "Longest Professional Wrestling Match." https://www.guinnessworldrecords.com/world-records/longest-match-professional-wrestling?.

Week 4
Luteal Phase: Who's Your Bible Mentor?

Watson, Stephanie. 2018. "Stages of the Menstrual Cycle," *Healthline*. https://www.healthline.com/health/womens-health/stages-of-menstrual-cycle#luteal.

Henry, Matthew. 1994. *Matthew Henry Study Bible-King James Version*. Nashville: Thomas Nelson, Inc., 1566.

Day 23
Fruitful in the Land of Affliction

Houston, Rickie. 2019. "Average Cost of Having a Baby in 2019." https://smart asset.com/financial-advisor/cost-of-having-a-baby.

"Cost of IVF: Cost Components." 2020. Fertility IQ. https://www.fertilityiq.com/ivf-in-vitro-fertilization/costs-of-ivf#cost-components.

Dasher, Eva. 2020. "First-Year Baby Costs Calculator," *Baby Center*, LLC. https://www.babycenter.com/baby-cost-calculator.

Day 24
Healing Tears

Gustafson, Timi. 2014. "Keeping Your Emotions Bottled Up Could Kill You," *Huffington Post*. https://www.huffingtonpost.ca/timi-gustafson/bottling-up-negative-emotions_b_5056433.html.

Day 26

Restoration of What Was Lost

Mayo Clinic. 2019. "Miscarriage." https://www.mayoclinic.org/diseases-conditions/ pregnancy-loss-miscarriage/symptoms-causes/syc-20354298.

About the Author

Reader. Writer. Builder. Follower of God. Author Kelli L. Ferguson has loved the written word for as long as she can remember. Working in the construction industry for over fifteen years has taught her the importance of making sure the foundation of a building is true. Just as a good foundation is critical to a building being structurally sound, having a good relationship with God is critical to a person being spiritually, emotionally, mentally, and physically well-formed. Her passion in life is to help women in their motherhood journey ensure that their foundations are built around God's Word.

Connect and Share

Did you enjoy *In the Meantime?* Please consider purchasing copies for women you know that may need inspiration during their conception journey. Be sure to leave a review on Amazon.com and BarnesandNoble.com.

Connect with Author Kelli L. Ferguson

Website: www.kellilferguson.com
Email: contact@kellilferguson.com
Instagram: @kellilferguson
Facebook: kellilferguson